BUSINESS ESSENTIALS FO

© 2018 Dr. Paul J. Pavlik
and
Tracker Enterprises, Inc.

Published by

Tracker Enterprises, Inc.
An Imprint of the Bija Company, LLC

1640 Pinnacle Ridge Lane
Colorado Springs, CO 80919
United States of America
www.trackerenterprises.com

ISBN 978-1-884059-27-8 (paperback)
ISBN 978-1-884059-28-5 (hardback)

First Printing

V 1.0

Printed in the United States of America.

DEDICATION

This book is dedicated to all of the honest, hard-working healthcare students, healthcare providers, practice owners and institutions who constantly labor at providing the absolute best products and services so that they can make life more enjoyable for the rest of us.

It is also dedicated to all of the business management authors, office managers, spouses, accountants, bookkeepers, financial advisors, bankers, and attorneys who work hard at trying to make healthcare professionals financially successful.

Most importantly, it's dedicated to our clients and viewers (all of whom we have come to call our close friends), with their vast combined experience and knowledge, who have given us countless insights into new ways of understanding the healthcare practice owner's needs.

*I respect all of you, and
I want you to be happy and successful.*

– Paul

ADVANCED PRAISE

BRAVO! Your book is such a helpful, informative and practical guide to all aspects of a healthcare career; it will definitely educate, inform, and provide a roadmap. It gives direction and helps to avoid, and/or prepare for the many potential potholes and detours over the years. This book will be an invaluable tool for all doctors.

- Kim Goehring, Healthcare Administrative & Management Coach

Dr. Pavlik's book is a masterpiece and treasure trove with valuable tips, insights, wisdom and processes for planning your life and business. It should be required reading for every healthcare professional. There is one paragraph on page 146 that makes the whole book worth more than a million dollars.

- Frank Candy, International Motivational Speaker & Author

As a student soon to graduate with a healthcare degree, entering the workforce and balancing clinical skills with the sudden pressure to obtain a wealth of knowledge about business and owning a practice can seem like a daunting task. Dr. Pavlik's book lays out beautifully the steps necessary to become a successful clinician – both as a business owner and in terms of quality patient care.

- Autumn Gray, Senior Dental Student

Dr. Pavlik's book is a valuable resource for years to come. I believe it is a great resource that will help guide students and recent graduates alike through a career in any health profession. This book is great for giving us an idea about the business side of dentistry – something that is briefly discussed while in school.

- Cody Jorgenson, Senior Dental Student

WOW!!! Your book is truly amazing. I realize your target audience, but there are many of us non-medical business folks who will gain great value from what you have written. I envision this being a book handed out at healthcare school graduations or being the #1 graduation gift for healthcare students around the world.

- Betsy Westhafer, CEO, The Congruity Group and Author

I sincerely enjoyed your book. In the past, I took several business courses in order to get an idea of what to expect in the business world. I found your book to be much easier to comprehend, engaging and not to mention, inspiring! I think it is a must-read for all healthcare professionals and especially for students like me who are unsure of what to do after graduation.

- Mariana Braga, Dental Student

What a wonderful gem! Every healthcare professional should have a copy. Paul has captured decades of experience and condensed it into an easy to use manual structured in a such a way that you can drop on any relevant topic and find expert informed opinion quickly. To find so much quality business information in one place is truly unique. Paul absolutely "gets it" and openly shares from the early stages in your career through Leadership, People, Financials and Exit Strategy. He will make you think about your life goals, business goals, patients and most importantly, yourself.

- Tony Bulleid
International Motivational & Coaching Expert
VP Sales, Marketing & Operations. EMEA

Although healthcare schools teach the skills necessary to work with patients, there is minimal to no business training. This book makes up for that and helps to uncover all the essential details to establish and eventually sell a successful practice, regardless of what stage the business is in. Dr. Pavlik has compiled a wealth of knowledge from his extensive healthcare experiences to provide practitioners with the fundamental tools to create a thriving practice. I highly recommend this book to any healthcare professional.

- Jordan New
Licensed Acupuncturist, MS Traditional Chinese Medicine

This book is awesome! I like the style – you address important topics in an engaging way, seeking to teach and explain rather than just direct. Every healthcare professional should find this educational and thought provoking.

- Mike Connolly, General Manager, TMP

WHAT OTHERS HAVE SAID

Dr. Paul Pavlik and his team from Tracker Enterprises is probably one of the most progressive financial and business building growth companies in the entire United States. Their attention to detail and complete understanding of financial issues surrounding growth is unsurpassed by anyone I know. They always take a great deal of time and genuine interest in truly knowing how to help a business grow and expand. They use their own knowledge and experience coupled with their proprietary business modeling software to assist healthcare businesses to truly capitalize on opportunity and provide the controls needed to sustain strong growth. It has always been a given that most businesses believe their CPA can do this kind of work and nothing could be further from the truth. It is important to have your CPA involved, but it takes an entirely different level of skills, experience and mindset to build success for the future. Tracker Enterprises possesses those skill sets and more. I think what I really like most about their group is they understand the subtle nuances associated with the expansion and growth issues of a business. I would recommend them to anyone.

R. C. S., President Axcelerate Worldwide, Inc.

I have been very pleased with the professional way my business affairs have been handled by Tracker. I particularly like the accessibility to Dr. Pavlik and his staff to bounce ideas off them, to forecast my financials, and to do what-if scenarios as they may pertain to different ways we may want to improve our business and financial reporting. Their efforts in analyzing my business have provided a great benefit to me during the transition of my business and, I am confident, will continue to provide the information and guidance to make my company more successful in the future."

R. G., President, Milwaukee, WI

It is very reassuring to know that I get REAL information to help me make important financial decisions. Tracker has also helped me in evaluations of staff members & showing them how their compensation effects overall production & expenses.

C. A., Office Manager

Great program & support team - the best I have been exposed to in my 20 plus years of practice. Accurately forecasting office trends is the key for success in today's clinical practice environment.

D. J. P., DC, President & CEO, AHC, Orlando, FL

We're a holistic practice & have been using Tracker for many years. Their financial analyses & forecasting along with monthly conferences have kept us competitive & financially healthy. Especially during these difficult economic times, these services are invaluable. What a mental relief it is to be able to anticipate & to prepare to deal with today's economic unpredictable turns. We would not be where we are today without Tracker.

Dr. G. E. V., DDS, Owner, CDM, Maine

Tracker helped maximize our productivity by way of their practice analysis tools & forecasting. Full staff analysis & training helped us meet our goals!

S. M. S., MD, Family Practice, Colorado Springs, CO

We are the largest chiropractic group practice in Central Florida & decided to see if all of our 5 clinics were making money. After Tracker detailed each of our centers, we were able to evaluate & make better financial decisions to help our company increase profits! Thanks.

A. K., Operations Manager, Orlando, FL

Over the past 3 years, our practice has worked with 2 dental consultants at a cost of $25,000. They were full of grandiose ideas. However, they lacked the one thing necessary to implement change: quantifiable results! Tracker helped us form a business plan. We learned how to run a practice as a business. Implementing the Tracker system has enabled our practice to increase production, lower costs, & maintain accounts receivable to a healthy ratio with production. Our practice has gone from survival to success to significance with Tracker.

Dr. J. L. H., DDS, President, CO

Tracker has been able to show us the financial health of our business. Reports are easy to understand, far superior to P&L statements. Tracker forecasts trends & prepares for changes we need to make to remain successful. We received a customized manual full of information prepared specifically for our business. Each month, Tracker meets with us to coach us on our financial decisions & track our progress. We can call Tracker anytime for advice; they're always available. We've had a great experience.

C. M., Office Manager, Denver, CO

We have used the services of Tracker Enterprises to enhance our ability to forecast the financial performance of our business. Dr. Pavlik and his team have made invaluable contributions to our recent success by not just giving us more detailed financial analysis than we could do ourselves, but also by helping us interpret the numbers to make positive changes to the daily operating aspects of the business resulting in increased revenues and better expense controls. The staff is engaging, knowledgeable, and always ready to be of assistance. In addition, it is fun to work with them!

M. J. C., Management, Vail, CO

"Tracker Enterprises has significantly helped our clients evaluate their current financial situation and plan for the future. This has helped place a successful timetable on their practice transitions."

P. K. S., Partner Practice Transitions, Denver, CO

As a financial consultant to a wide range of practices, working with the team at Tracker Enterprises has been a major success for the our company. Many of our clients have benefited from the forecasting and projecting expertise provided by Tracker Enterprises. This has resulted in a positive financial impact by returning our clients to a bankable position and enabling us to provide the necessary financial funding for daily operations.

M. R. C., CEO, Consulting Group, CO

Very informative. Education is the key to success. Tracker was extremely helpful. Thanks for your help.

K. L., Vice President, Colorado Springs, CO

We have been using Tracker Enterprises to forecast expense and revenue trends for months and years ahead. Tracker's unique program and coaching allow me, on a moment's notice, to successfully adjust to the current dynamically changing business environment. Their team is always available for my questions. Finally, I am able to accurately predict where my business will be tomorrow and well into the future. Best of all, my bottom line continues to improve. Thank you, Tracker Enterprises.

M. C. V., President, Pittsburgh, PA

With 35 years experience, I was continually struggling just to maintain financial status quo. Enlisting the services of Tracker Enterprises was the smartest decision I have made in my business career. Through their guidance and support systems, my business now thrives and I am free to concentrate on what I do best.

M. B., Owner, CO

I recently purchased a practice. Dr. Paul Pavlik represented the buyer in the sale. Nonetheless, as the purchaser, I received helpful information and coaching from Dr. Pavlik that made my decision to purchase very simple. He provided detailed reports that reassured me that I was making a wise purchase. Additionally, Dr. Pavlik was always available to answer questions throughout the process. His knowledge and expertise were invaluable.

Dr. AP, Bangor, ME

Thank you again for your very detailed response. You have no idea how much I appreciate someone with your wealth of industry knowledge providing such useful feedback concerning my situation. People like you make this an amazing industry to be a part of.

Dr. M.V, SC

The service & information provided by Tracker is exceptional. The information is easily visualized & the ability to rapidly do retro & prospective research of practice financial parameters is unique.

Dr. R. W., DDS, President, HDC, Denver, CO

READER'S GUIDE – BOOK ORGANIZATION

This book is a guide on how the healthcare professional might address the business life cycles that all of us experience. I discuss leadership first, however, since without proper leadership skills, it will be difficult to manage business at any stage of your career. Sections II through V address the business life cycles. Section VI discusses what someone who wants to be an employee should expect. The end of each section contains a **Summary** and a **Road Map** to show where you are in your journey.

Each Section is introduced with a story about my personal journey. Then, I discuss business knowledge every healthcare professional should have and what to do to obtain these skills.

Although my goal is to have you read the entire book, it's okay to jump to chapters (see Table of Contents) that pertain to a particular time in your career you want to address.

Italicized Quotes & Illustrations

Quotes and illustrations are used to inspire you to read on, to emphasize a point I am trying to make, or simply to have fun. Caricatures are meant to represent me throughout my career.

Text Boxes

Text boxes further describe the subject being discussed in the main text.

A, b, c

I have tried to cover every subject from your education through the end of your healthcare career. This book is definitely not the last word. At the end of each section, you will be prompted to further your knowledge and/or how to contact me to discuss your thoughts and goals. Please get in touch and stay in touch.

X, y, z

TABLE OF CONTENTS

Dedication...iii

Advanced Praise...iv

What Others Have Said...vi

Reader's Guide – Book Organization...x

Disclaimer... xviii

Acknowledgements xix

Foreword... xx

Introduction Do Not Skip Ahead - Read This First! 5

Are You Experiencing a Crisis? 7

Who Should Read This Book?...8

This book is for every healthcare professional including:........8

This book addresses every stage of your career: 8

If you own your practice, why did you start it?...........................8

Where Are You in Your Business Life Cycle?...........................9

What's My Responsibility To You?...10

What's the Point?..11

Section I: The Art of a Leader 15

Chapter 1: First, A Few Interesting Stories to Share...........15

Leadership Scenario 1: Remember the Golden Rule...............15

Leadership Scenario 2: Don't lead from a podium 16

Chapter 2: Make Yourself a Leader.....................................18

The new age of leadership 18

Who is responsible?...19

What is the secret to having great employees? 20

The Ideal Performance Management Process..............................20

Pump up employee enthusiasm 22

An effective employee performance review system.................23

Domination is unacceptable 26

The leadership paradox..27

Chapter 3: What's really important?...............................28

You're in the people business 28

Listen, listen, and then, listen 29

Chapter 4: The Mutual Fussiness Factor................................30

Chapter 5: When Staff Members Resist....................................31

Chapter 6: Employee Handbooks..32

What to include in an Employee Handbook..............................33

Sample of Employee Handbook Table of Contents...................35

Chapter 7: When It's Time to Part Ways 39

When is it time to move on?..39

Do you need to give a reason for employee dismissal?..........40

Section I: Summary & Leadership Action Plan.....................42

Section II: Launch 45

Chapter 8: My Story Begins With My Launch.......................45

Phase 1: The long preparation 45

Phase 2: Spending time on the couch 45

Chapter 9: How To Launch Your Career..................................49

You graduated – now what?...49

Eventually, you will have to understand business 50

Chapter 10: Will You Be a Small Business? 51

Will your practice be considered a small business?................51

Why is your small business so important?......................................51

Challenges & Risks..52

Why Do Practices Fail?...52

Chapter 11: How To Start Your Practice?..............................55

What about the money you will need?..55

What's the approval rate for small business loans?...................56

What is the average time to get funding?.....................................56

What type of healthcare service do you provide?.......................56

What business structure should you choose?..............................57

How to start the planning process 58

Do you need a business plan?...58

A typical Business Plan will include:...59

Your advisory staff and what you should expect? 63

Section II: Summary & Launch Action Plan 64

Section III: Expand...67

Chapter 12: My Story Continues - Expanding.......................67

Chapter 13: Your Story Continues - Expanding....................69

Does a healthcare degree guarantee success? 69

Are you immune to understanding business?..............................69

Do you need to have a business background?...............................71

How do you rank yourself?..71

Do you need to understand financial statements? 71

Where do you want to go with your business?............................72

Can you guarantee success? 72

Consider these questions:...73

Right now, you are probably making excuses 73

Thinking it through 74

Know your 3 Ws: 75

Chapter 14: The Genesis of Your Practice 77

What is your job description? 77

Growing pains 78

The point of no return 80

There is another way ... .81

Chapter 15: Understanding Financial Reports...................83

First, do you speak the language? 83

Second, do you understand the script............................87

If you don't have the info, you can't make the decisions 96

You need a system 97

Section III: Summary & Expand Action Plan 98

Section IV: Optimize... 101

Chapter 16: My Story Continues To Improve..................... 101

Chapter 17: Your Story - Take the Right Path................... 105

What is the optimal model to manage your practice? 107

The Ingredients to Optimal Operational Management.........108

What do you need to make smart financial decisions? 110

What would this Optimal Management tool look like? 113

Chapter 18: Who Needs A Budget, Anyway? 115

What is a Budget?...116

Why should you consider a budget for your practice?.........117

Making budget estimates 117

Reasons for budgeting 118

A budget has these additional advantages: 119

There are two ways to budget from year to year:...............119

Why some practices avoid budgeting 120

The importance of detailed budgets 120

Information you will need to prepare a budget 121

Hierarchy of budgeting 124

Sample Healthcare Professional Budget 126

Chapter 19: Forecasting - The Real Game-Changer..........129

What exactly is a forecast?...............................130

What's the difference between budgets and forecasts?.......130

Forecasting is the basis for planning.........................130

Hierarchy of forecasting 131

Forecasting methodologies 132

Reasons for forecasting 133

Sample Actuals & Forecasts 135

Sample Written Analysis of Actuals and Forecasts 136

Make forecasting a habit; you won't regret it. 137

Section IV: Summary & Optimize Action Plan...................138

Section V: Sell...141

Chapter 20: My Story Continues With a Surprise 141

Chapter 21: You - Prepare an End Game Plan..................143

When to prepare an Exit Plan.............................143

How to start preparing an Exit Plan 143

How long should Exit Planning take? 144

Do Exit Plans evolve?......................................144

When is the best time to sell?..............................145

Are you really in touch with your future? 146

Do you have a plan? 146

What are some exit planning excuses? 147

Is exit planning worth it? 148

When should you start exit planning? 149

Will there be a market for your practice? 149

What else should you consider? 150

Start with the end in mind 151

Protect yourself and your family 151

Where can you find potential buyers? 153

Why setting goals is important, even if they change 153

Chapter 22: Introduction to the Valuation 155

What you should initially provide to a potential buyer? 155

The practice valuation generally should also include 156

How to arrive at a value for the practice ... .157

Valuation methods typically used ... .158

Valuation criteria to consider 159

Minimum items needed to evaluate a practice 160

Detailed valuation items you will want to know 160

Chapter 23: How to Increase Practice Value 162

What Are Value Drivers? 162

Why Value Drivers Matter 163

Benefits of Value Drivers: 163

Business models for exit strategy planning 164

Chapter 24: Should You Consider an HSO? 166

Chapter 25: How Involved is the Selling Process 169

Selling Process Overview 170

Things you need to remember 172

All goals must be SMART 173

Both buyer and seller have goals 173

Do You Need an Attorney? 174

The provisions of the deal 175

Section V: Summary & Sell Action Plan 176

Section VI: Should You Work for Someone Else? 179

Chapter 26: Employment Options 179

Chapter 27: Relationship Concerns 180

What to consider before becoming an employee 180

What can ruin an associate/owner relationship 181

Chapter 28: Understanding the Associate Contract 182

Chapter 29: Independent Contractor – Beware 191

Understand the definitions first 191

Advantages to Employers and Contractors 192

Disadvantages for Independent Contractors 193

How the IRS defines an Independent Contractor 193

The consequences of misclassifying workers 195

Chapter 30: Does Renting Space Make Sense? 197

Section VI: Summary & Employment Action Plan 198

Section VII: In a Nutshell 200

Postscript 207

Bibliography 210

About the Author 214

Caricature Illustrations By 216

DISCLAIMER

Neither the author nor publisher assumes responsibilities for errors, inaccuracies, or omissions. The information contained in this publication is general in nature and is not intended for use as a source of security, technical, legal, accounting, financial, or other professional advice. For information regarding your particular situation, contact an attorney or a tax or financial advisor. In specific cases, clients should consult their legal, accounting, tax or financial advisor. This book is not intended to give advice or to represent me or my firm as being qualified to give advice in all areas of professional services. To the extent that the author or the firm does not have the expertise required on a particular matter, we will always work closely with you to help you gain access to the resources and professional advice that you need.

Neither the author nor the publisher accepts any responsibility or liability for your use of the ideas presented herein. Conversely, neither the publisher nor author will lay claim to any profits you make based on the suggestions of this book.

Some suggestions made in this book concerning business practices may have inadvertently introduced practices deemed unlawful in certain states, municipalities, or countries. You should be aware of the various laws governing your business practices in your particular industry and in your location.

Any slights of people or organizations are unintentional.

While the Web sites referenced were personally reviewed by the author, there are no guarantees to their safety or accuracy. These sources were referenced with all due respect for the authors. Practice safe Internet surfing with current antivirus software and a browser with active security settings. All photos, images, charts, graphs, etc. were provided either through copyright approval by Tracker Enterprises, Inc. or through Google Advanced Image Search with approval for "free to use or share or modify, even commercially" at
https://www.google.com/advanced_image_search

ACKNOWLEDGEMENTS

Special thanks to Beverly, my wife and CFO (both Chief Financial Officer and "Chief Fun Officer"), for giving me confidence in believing we have something unique and important to offer, for putting up with my absence during the research and writing of this book, and for her continuing support and expert advice. She deserves an achievement award for her continued editing, excellent suggestions and recommendations throughout all of the versions and drafts of this book.

Thanks to Aimee Haywood, my daughter, for sharing her experiences as an author, and for being my advisor and friend. Thanks to Chris Haywood, my son-in-law, for his spiritual guidance and for telling me I had it in me to persevere through the writing of this book.

Thanks to Paul Michael Pavlik, my son, for keeping me on track, giving me spiritual guidance, and being my fly-fishing buddy and music mentor. Thanks to Erin Pavlik, my daughter-in-law, for giving me the confidence in my teaching skills to persevere.

Extra thanks to Gary Carpenter (a true friend and very smart man), whose brain melded perfectly with mine in conceiving and developing the software we use and the concepts we teach.

Thanks to Frank Candy, a new and dear friend, who has, for no other reason than offering his friendship and expertise, made great suggestions for teaching me how to attract and then keep an audience.

A very special thanks to Mark S. A. Smith who has been giving me more help than any friend should be expected to do, and who has given me the encouragement, guidance and especially for his mentorship to complete this book and for teaching me how to enjoy life more.

FOREWORD

You've made an important decision in choosing this book. You've decided that to be a successful healer, you must have a business operation that's healthy. There are no patients to treat when there's no clinic, staff, equipment, or financially sound doctor.

Your ability to have a profitable, sustainable, scalable, and ultimately salable practice means that you're not concerned about your personal welfare or that of your team, therefore you can devote your entire cognitive capacity to solving and preventing the health issues of your patient. Isn't this why you studied so long and hard?

The bottom line, you can't be a great doctor when you're concerned about your financial wellbeing. When you carefully apply this book's concepts, you complete your training in that you know how to operate a clinic that cures patients and commensurately compensates you for it.

"Doctors concerned for their own wealth cannot be focused on their patients' health."

Your mentor in this is Dr. Paul Pavlik, a thoughtful, intelligent doctor with a history of a successful practice, and more importantly, a history of coaching many doctors to enjoy a profitable practice. This book is the distillation of his decades of business experience applied to the world of healthcare, navigating and weathering political and economic storms.

I'm honored to know Dr. Paul for more than two decades. He is a man of impeccable integrity, with a careful and thoughtful approach to medicine and business, a talented musician, and a valued friend. You're fortunate to have his attention and access his wisdom.

Here's the good news, you can become a better than average business person under the guidance of Dr. Paul. It will take you a small fraction of the time to accomplish this compared with if you had to figure it out on your own, making mistakes, and paying the "stupid tax". Oh, we all pay it if we choose to strike out on our own. No need to, business acumen is well defined, and Dr. Paul is a master.

"Find advisors whose history is your future.
Ignore everyone else's advice."

Make this commitment to yourself: invest what's required to put into practice what you've worked so hard to master. Give your business development the time, thought, and money that it needs to support you for the rest of your life. To sell yourself short as a business owner is to disrespect your professors, your patients, and your hard work mastering your art.

"The more that you're a financial success,
the more that your patients will
experience healing success."

With your financial success, you will change your world. Are you ready for the adventure?

Let's go!

Mark S. A. Smith
Business Growth Strategist
Author, consultant, speaker, podcaster
BijaCo.com

Imagine how satisfying your professional journey can be if you have a definite plan throughout each of your business life cycles.

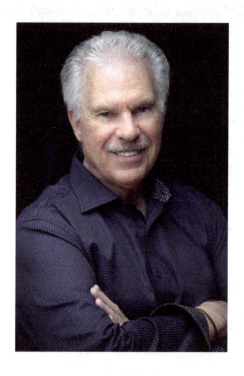

My goal is to make your journey as stress-free and successful as possible.

- Dr. Paul J. Pavlik

Business Essentials

for Healthcare Professionals

How to Operate a Sustainable,

Profitable, and Salable Practice

or Successfully Work for Someone Else

Dr. Paul J. Pavlik

*A goal without a plan
is just a wish.*
Antoine de Saint-Exupery

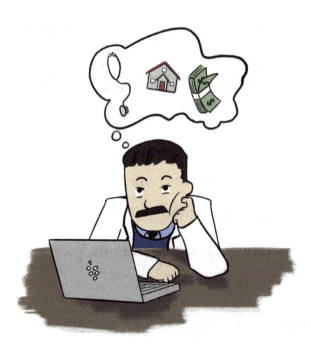

INTRODUCTION
DO NOT SKIP AHEAD - READ THIS FIRST!

Healthcare professionals often struggle with the business aspect of their practices. Part of the reason why is because all businesses go through life cycles just like humans do.

Whether you're preparing for a career, or launching a practice, or growing a practice, or making your practice the best it can be, or getting ready to sell your practice, what you do in each one of those business life cycles is very different. We don't get taught how to deal with those in school.

I work with healthcare professionals, wherever they happen to be in their business life cycle, to help them achieve success in that stage and future stages of their practices.

The goal is to be comfortable with the business of your practice, predictable with your cash flows, and to have money in your bank accounts. And ultimately, to be able to sell your practice to the right person for the most you possibly can.

This book provides a road map for your professional career and guidelines to better understand the business of your practice. It takes the power away from dwelling in the past, where none of us has the ability to undo what was done no matter who is to blame. It's a constructive effort. Everyone wants to succeed, but few are willing to pay the price. You don't determine your future; you determine your habits, and your habits determine your future. The secret lies in developing a routine of understanding the business of your business, doing it on a regular basis and then acting on what you see.

Expect the best. Prepare for the worst.
Capitalize on what comes.

Zig Ziglar

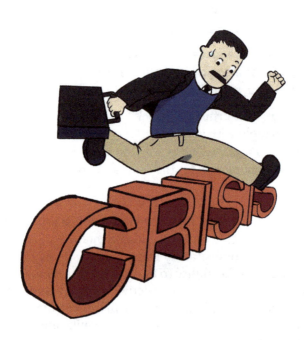

Are You Experiencing a Crisis?

As healthcare professionals, we are more likely to define a **crisis** as a turning point for better or worse in a patient's acute disease process (e.g., fever, etc.) or a dangerous time or event in which a solution is needed quickly (e.g., serious traumatic injury).[1]

Another way of defining a crisis is that it can be a significant or unstable event, a turning point, or a radical change of status in your personal or business life by which the trend of all future events is determined. If not handled in an appropriate and timely manner, it may turn into a catastrophe for your business.[2] This is the definition we should welcome since crisis can then initiate action and improvement.

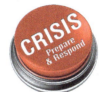

No matter what stage of the Business Life Cycle (Launch, Expand, Optimize, Sell) you are currently experiencing, you are constantly exposed to some type of crisis situation, whether it be a new situation that needs addressing immediately, or whether you are transitioning from one stage of your Life Cycle to another.

People going through crisis need to adjust to new and unfamiliar circumstances. You may be feeling overwhelmed, so this book is meant to help you sort out how to better understand the financial issues. This book invites you to understand your business concerns and then suggests another way of looking at things. You need to be able to focus on what is important and then give it immediate attention. Instead of rehashing the past and worrying about how that might affect your future, past experiences should encourage you to concentrate on and improve the present. Then, rather than being paralyzed by the past, by better understanding the present, you will prepare yourself to properly deal with your future and make it a successful journey.

---

[1] https://www.dictionary.com/browse/crisis

[2] https://www.merriam-webster.com/dictionary/crisis

WHO SHOULD READ THIS BOOK?

This book is for every healthcare professional including:

- Dentists
- Medical physicians
- Osteopathic physicians
- Chiropractors
- Veterinary physicians
- Military doctors
- Other ancillary healthcare providers and office managers
- Students studying for a degree in the healthcare professions
- Healthcare professionals already employed or wanting to be employed by someone else

This book addresses every stage of your career:

- Still studying to be a healthcare provider,
- In the military trying to decide what to do next,
- Hired as an associate in another practice,
- Thinking of starting your own practice,
- Working as an office manager trying to improve the practice,
- Working as an ancillary professional (therapist, etc.),
- Just getting started in your own private practice,
- Making the most of your existing practice, or
- Considering a transition out of practice.

If you own your practice, why did you start it?

- Have a passion to help people get healthier and then help them to stay healthy.
- Like to control everything.
- Had a great idea for making money.
- No one else would employ you.
- It's your definition of freedom and controlling your destiny.

WHERE ARE YOU IN YOUR BUSINESS LIFE CYCLE?

You are in or will be in one of the following stages of your professional life cycle or transitioning between stages:

1. **Launch** – just starting or considering your career.
2. **Expand** – in practice, but wanting to grow.
3. **Optimize** – wanting to be the best provider you can be.
4. **Sell** – considering a transition out of practice.

Each life cycle of your practice is aimed at focusing on the strategies necessary to exit your practice in style:

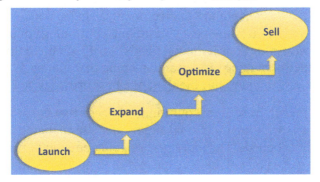

©Tracker Enterprises, Inc. 2018

Regardless of the business life cycle you and your practice are experiencing, this book should provide you with valuable information that will help you reach or exceed your goals.

Since studying business can often seem tedious, at best, to healthcare professionals who prefer to concentrate their efforts in a clinical environment, I will try to make this book more interesting by introducing each Section with a story that relates to either my own personal experience or to the experiences of other healthcare professionals I have had the privilege to know. The references may be real or fictionalized to make the lessons learned more impactful, but **the value is real**. After each of the stories, you will discover a basic understanding of business and how its principles can be used by any healthcare professional.

9

WHAT'S MY RESPONSIBILITY TO YOU?

Since I went into the healthcare profession because I wanted to help others in need of my knowledge and clinical skills, since I have walked the walk of a healthcare provider, and since I have worked with all types of healthcare providers, regardless of their disciplines, from single practitioner practices with two employees up to 600 employee surgical centers, I can relate to your needs and concerns. I know you want to be the best provider you can be to obtain the best outcome for your patients, but *you must be financially successful* to do these things. And, whether you admit it or not, success means making enough money to pay for a good location, a pleasant clinical environment, a skilled and compassionate staff, the best equipment, continuing education and providing for your personal needs. So, if I allude to the importance of making money and keeping that money, it is because I want you to be able to be the best provider you can be.

It is my job to address four kinds of needs that every business owner has including functional, emotional, life changing and social impact needs. The more of these elements that I provide to you, the more you will believe me and then put the content to use.

1. **Social impact** – Outcomes make life better for everyone including you, your family, your staff and, most importantly, your customers (i.e., your patients).
2. **Life changing** – The concepts presented should make your business life easier and your practice more productive and thus, make your personal life more rewarding and enjoyable.
3. **Emotional** – The goals are to reduce anxiety, provide access to the previously unknown, and be of value.
4. **Functional** – The system saves time, simplifies life, makes money, reduces risk, organizes, integrates, connects, reduces effort, reduces costs, improves quality and informs.[3]

---

[3] Bain & Company, 2015, *The Elements of Value*, September 2016

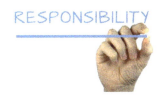

RESPONSIBILITY

I understand that ...

1. It's not your fault that you may not have a thorough grasp of business acumen. Finance and business education courses are rare, if given at all, in the current healthcare universities and the professional curriculums they offer.
2. I need to be able to show you the basic financial knowledge you need to demonstrate how your business works or should work without adding more time to your busy schedule. You should be spending your non-clinical time staying up with current trends and continuing education and having more opportunities to spend time with your family.

Since everyone is a skeptic, I have to be able to answer questions:

1. Why am I bothering you with this material?
2. Why should you care?
3. Why should you believe me?
4. Why should you do anything going forward?

WHAT'S THE POINT?

With all of the professional journals and other scientific literature you receive and need to read on a regular basis to stay current, why would you possibly want to read about how to interpret your financial statements and how those financials have an impact on the operations of your practice? Why would you want to spend time thinking about retiring from your practice when you are just getting started? In addition, with all of the certified public accountants, financial advisors, attorneys, management software, and business books currently available, it would seem that all that needs to be said about understanding the finances of your practice has been said.

Maybe you ...

- Are still searching for something that not only helps you understand what your financials are trying to tell you but also helps you plan for the future.
- Need to know how to react to the ever-changing financial environment as it attempts to throw you off the path to success.
- Are looking for some help in understanding your financials without having to be a financial wizard – some technique that lets you understand the numbers as they apply to your practice, not someone else's practice.
- Would rather spend, at most, no more than an hour each month understanding your financials instead of days, or worse, not understanding them at all.

Well, there is better way – a method that should be considered *as an adjunct, not a replacement*, to all of the experts and the tools mentioned above. This philosophy is the method we referred to earlier called **Business Life Cycle Management**. The idea of Business Life Cycle Management may be new to you, but this system will be discussed frequently as you continue through the book.

So, if you want to understand how to make the money that will allow you to provide great service to your patients and enjoy a wonderful life style, this book offers the resources to continue to do good for your patients, yourself and all of those around you.

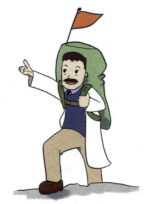

OK, *let's start the journey* ...

Ignorance is not bliss.

You are the person you've been looking for –
no one else is coming!
If you're willing to accept responsibility for your life,
you'll discover that no matter what
other people do or don't do,
you're accountable to yourself.
You decide how to respond.
You decide to continue to move
toward your dreams, or not.
Prince Charming isn't waiting around the next corner;
your ship isn't coming in.
The odds are against you winning the lottery.

So what are you going to do?

You can do one of two things:
die at the gate of complaint, or
take the responsibility and emerge
with a strategy that enables you to succeed.

Take the temperature for your life and
change the terms for your future.

A leader is one who KNOWS the way, GOES the way, and SHOWS the way.

John C. Maxwell

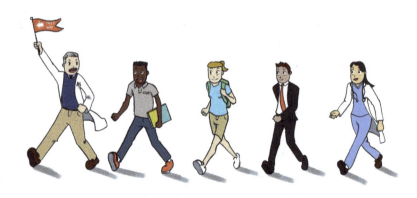

SECTION I: THE ART OF A LEADER

CHAPTER 1: A FEW INTERESTING STORIES TO SHARE

A company can only go as fast as the leader goes!
Mark S. A. Smith

In the Introduction, I indicated that I would start off each section with either a personal story about myself or a story about other healthcare professionals who have shared their experiences. The following Leadership experiences are scenarios about other healthcare professionals I know; their experiences have been altered to protect their identities. As you might imagine, I have several other examples regarding questionable leadership, but the following will be enough to show you the universal need to develop excellent leadership skills.

Leadership Scenario 1: Remember the Golden Rule

Scenario:

This doctor had a leadership approach that was "authoritarian" to say the least. He thought of himself as being beyond intellectual questioning and above reproach. Therefore, when he dealt with employees who were not living up to his expectations, he admonished them in front of the other staff and patients. He also had no concept of time and therefore was consistently late for patients without offering an excuse. Although he had staff meetings, he frequently ran over into patients' scheduled appointments and never apologized. He was consistently behind (often over a month) in doing chart entries and dictation; yet, he publicly criticized his insurance department for not collecting on accounts (these accounts had never been submitted to insurance or billed to patients since he had been delinquent about entering the treatment or the treatment codes in the day sheets).

Leadership Error:

This doctor had no respect for anyone but himself. Although his employees were trying to accomplish what they thought he expected, they were guessing at best since he had never coached them regarding his preferred treatment methods, and they had no written guidelines to follow, e.g., an Employee Handbook. He expected them to "automatically" know everything based on their past experience and education. He never met with them to discuss their progress and therefore, they never knew how they were doing. This was the typical bad leader approach of the "leave alone – ZAP" methodology.

A leader must lead by example. If he expected promptness, he needed to be on time. No staff should be asked to deal with irate patients because the doctor lacked respect or personal discipline.

A leader curates and then enforces the culture of the practice.

Leadership Scenario 2: Don't lead from a podium

Scenario:

This doctor had a beautiful practice and a great location. Aside from production not being at the level he expected, he was losing staff because they were frustrated with him. Making appointments was difficult for the patients because his schedule was booked well into the future, but several holes developed daily in the schedule. He blamed this on the staff for not communicating well enough with the patients, yet he had never trained them to do so. In addition, patients had to be rescheduled because he ran over on his appointments.

Leadership Error:

Staff meetings were held frequently, but the owner/doctor took complete control, and blamed the staff for every other problem in the office. He also spoke to them from behind a barrier (elevated desk, i.e., a podium, front of the room, etc.) and never gave them a chance to respond or make suggestions. He never gave the staff a written or verbal roadmap so that they could aim at the destination he desired. Remember that two or more brains are always better than one

These are only a few examples. As I will state over and over again, healthcare professionals rarely, if ever, receive business training as part of their healthcare education. This lack of the education needed to operate a business with sound business principles also applies to the lack of leadership education. Without leadership skills, how can a provider ever expect to get the results desired, have the respect of the staff, and be capable of self-guidance throughout that provider's business and personal life cycles?

> *Profit is the applause you get*
> *for taking care of your customers and*
> *creating a motivating environment for your people.*
> Ken Blanchard

The following tells you nearly everything you need to know to have a great practice experience:

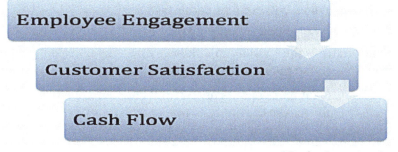

©Tracker Enterprises, Inc.

No practice, small or large, can win over the long run without energized employees who believe in the mission and understand how to achieve it. [4]

This section is an obvious tie-in to what will be discussed in this book going forward. <u>If you're going to succeed, your team has to be behind you</u>. So, read on for a little bit of leadership advice.

---

4 Jack Welch, former CEO of General Electric

CHAPTER 2: MAKE YOURSELF A LEADER

The new age of leadership ...

Although my emphasis in this book will be about how important it is for you to understand your expenses and profitability and how to prepare for continued success in your career, I want to spend a little time on how vital your employees are in your realization of success. Unfortunately, in today's world, the norm has become putting a misplaced emphasis on reports and statistics rather than on people. The leadership you represent sets the frame for the rest of this book. You need to declare: "*I am the leader*." Declaring is a great first step, but declaration is not enough. **You actually have to be a leader** and you must be a good one. Understand that leadership is second in importance only to your license to practice. Now, let's explore a small sampling of how you can be a better leader.

The new age definition for leadership is as follows: **Leadership** is the capacity to influence others by unleashing their power and potential to impact the greater good.[5]

If you want more out of yourself and your employees, you have to truly believe the quote, "*None of us is as smart as all of us.*" No matter how much you know and how experienced you are, adding additional IQ, experience and passion to the mix increases your chances for success. Every employee has something valuable to offer.

Now, consider Ken Blanchard's definition of a team: "A **team** is two or more persons who come together for a common purpose and who are mutually accountable for results."

Do you now see the importance of phrases like "*impact the greater good,*" "*come together for a common purpose*" and "*mutually responsible for results*"? These phrases are all commonalities for exceptional teams and leaders.

---

[5] Blanchard, Carlos, & Randolph. Empowerment Takes More Than a Minute·

Who is responsible?

Think about this:

1. If you want to know why your people are not performing well, step up to the mirror and take a peek, and conversely,
2. If you want to know why your people are performing well, step up to the mirror and take a peek.

The mirror I am talking about has room enough for only one individual -- YOU. You are the owner, and therefore, you are the master leader. Step up to that mirror and be counted and measured.

You know that you are the owner of your practice, and therefore, you carry the ultimate responsibility for its success. You know (or should know) your goals and what is needed to accomplish those goals. Do your employees know anything or, better yet, everything about your goals and visions? Every owner also wants the employees to take ownership for their responsibilities. Why then, do so many owners forget to give employees the tools needed to make for a more successful outcome and a better work environment? Usually, it is because the owner believes the employees should know their jobs intuitively and then, that owner does not care or does not know how to coach their employees.

Understand this:

"People without information cannot act responsibly."

Then, it must follow that:

"People with information are compelled to act responsibly."

What is the secret to having great employees?

Your employees don't care how much you know until they know how much you care.
Damon Richards

Doctor/owners often assume they can go about their day, work hard, be nice to their employees, and then assume, because of the employees' past training and experience that the employees will automatically know what to do. YOU need to train them how YOU want things done. If you cut your employees loose without any direction, they will lose their way, and your practice will suffer immeasurably.

> If those you are leading don't know where you are going, they will have a hard time getting excited about the journey.

The man who walks in the dark does not know where he is going.

The Ideal Performance Management Process

When you want to start off right with a new employee or start off on a "new leaf" with an existing employee, try this:

1. **Find out** from them exactly what they do know.
2. **Tell them** exactly what you want them to do. Even if they have been highly trained and/or are coming from a previous job, never expect them to know what you want exactly.
3. Even if you think they know or if they think they know what you want, **teach them** what you want them to do – exactly.
4. **Observe them** doing the task.
5. **Praise them** when they get anything right.
6. **Redirect and retrain** in the areas they are not getting right.
7. Continue to **praise them** for any progress, frequently.
8. **Tell them** how you will monitor and measure their progress.
9. **Monitor and measure their progress** on a regular basis.
10. **Meet with them** often to praise and redirect (not once/year at their annual review); meet no less than once/month.

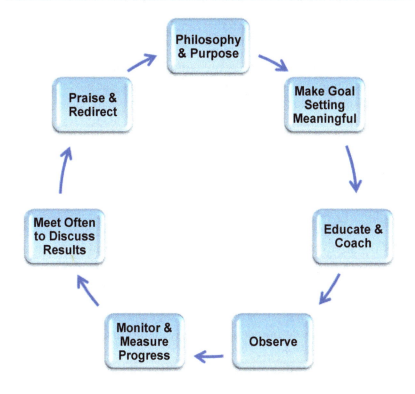

©Tracker Enterprises, Inc. 2018

Treat them as if they were full partners (i.e., be transparent with your measurements of their progress mentioned above), and they will take ownership of their responsibilities. When you think of your people as partners, they take responsibility for what they do, and that is exactly what you want them to do. *This means you have to show them why you are monitoring and measuring their performance and then give them the tools and training they need to succeed, and show them the targets they need to aim at for success.*

Set clear goals, then observe and measure performance.
Follow by praising progress, even minimal progress,
and redirect inappropriate behavior.

Pump up employee enthusiasm ...

Keep in mind that your employees are your practice's greatest assets. Their ideas, feedback, and enthusiasm for what they do can help your practice grow and succeed. Some people are naturally wired to give their all and do their best no matter where they work, but the majority of people require the guidance of skilled leaders who welcome their ideas, ask for feedback, and generate enthusiasm in order to give employees a sense of purpose and energy about what they do.

1. **Start by letting go of any negative opinions** you may have about your employees. Approach each of them as a source of unique knowledge with something valuable (positive or negative) to contribute to your practice. Remember, you are co-creating the vision with them. Positive feedback is fulfilling, but even negative feedback can guide you on what not to do. Get to know your employees, especially their goals, what stresses them in their job, what excites them, and how each of them defines success. Show an interest in their well-being and do what it takes.

2. **Make sure your employees** have everything they need to do their jobs. Ask each staff member, "*Do you have everything you need to be as competent as you can be?*"

3. **Clearly communicate what is expected**, what your values and visions are, and how you define success. Employees cannot perform well or be productive if they do not know what it is they are there to do and the part they play in your practice's success. Communicate your expectations, give them goals, measure progress, and show them how they have done -- and do it often.

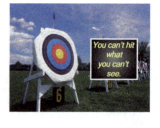

4. **Make sure your employees are trained**, retrained, and retrained again in problem solving and communication skills. These critical skills will help them interact better with you, their co-workers, suppliers, and most importantly, the customers (patients).

5. **Constantly ask how you are doing** in your employees' eyes. It can be difficult to request employee feedback, and it can be equally, if not more difficult, for an employee to give the person who evaluates them an honest response. To develop this skill and model it for your employees, begin dialogues with employees using such conversation starters as, "*It is one of my goals to constantly improve myself as a doctor and employer. What would you like to see me do differently? What could I be doing to make your job easier?*" Be sure to accept feedback graciously, express appreciation, and then, act on their recommendations, if appropriate.

6. **Pay attention to employee interactions**. Do they repeat stories of success or stories of shame? Stay away from participating in discussions that are destructive. On the other hand, do not hesitate to keep success stories alive and well.

7. **Reward and recognize** employees in ways meaningful to them. Celebrate your employees' accomplishments and efforts to work on achieving your and their goals.

8. **Be consistent**. If you ask employees to start an initiative and then you drop it, your efforts will backfire creating employee confusion. There is a connection between an employee's commitment to an initiative and a leader's commitment to supporting it. Your ongoing commitment to keeping your staff engaged, involved, and excited about the work they do and the challenges they face <u>must be a daily priority</u>.[6]

An effective employee performance review system

First, it is assumed that you, as the owner/leader, already have a component in your Employee Handbook (more on Employee Handbooks later in this section) that indicates when, how often, and what is covered in a "performance review." If you do not have an official review system in place, PREPARE ONE NOW.

Giving a "grade" on employees' progress since their last review should never be a once-per-year occurrence. Your

---

[6] Brandi, JoAnna.

employees need more frequent feedback as to their progress and improvement. Setting goals and criticizing performance once per year will have a great amount of impact on your employees at the time of the review (e.g., fear of being viewed as incompetent, fear of being stupid, fear of missing out on a decent raise, etc.). Doing reviews infrequently will result in discussions that are quickly forgotten, implied goals that, over time, may stray off of your desired path, or worse, allow them to think that since you only discuss the problems once per year, you give minimal importance to subjects discussed in the reviews!

Leave Alone – ZAP!!!

Don't be a "**Leave alone – ZAP**" boss; i.e., don't let employee issues stew until the annual review and then tell them you are unhappy with their performance because of this issue, that issue, blah, blah, blah! Showing frequent interest in your employees will make them feel better about themselves.

By consistently monitoring, praising, mentoring, teaching, and redirecting, your employees receive reinforcement toward the results you desire and constant redirection when they stray.

Teacher, how can I get an "A"?

When you went to school, regardless of the grade level, did you, your parents and your teachers aspire to a goal for you of getting all A's -- or, were B's, C's, D's, and F's an acceptable end-result? I am not saying that some of us realized, at some point in our education, that we did not have the ability, interest, or desire in certain subjects to always believe that an "A" was possible or necessary. What I am saying is that if our teachers had given us all of the information needed to pass every test (i.e., the teachers gave us proper information for every test question in advance), would it not be realistic to believe that most of us would have received A's on every test and semester grades? Would our chances for future success have increased? What do you think?

Why then, do we, as leaders, feel we can tell our employees what is expected of them, ask them to do the required tasks, and then, LEAVE THEM ALONE? (e.g., for a year)? Why do we expect good performance and results when we don't tell them in advance what good performance and results are? Moreover, do we assume that they know how to teach themselves without any guidance and training from us (the experts)? Why do we wait a year since the last performance review to give them a "grade" when we don't periodically review their performance (i.e., test and grade them more frequently) and then, redirect their efforts? Most importantly, why do we criticize their efforts (grade them below an "A") when, had we trained them properly (given them the information in advance), they could have the tools to perform admirably so that your business runs ideally – isn't that what you, your employees, and ultimately, your patients really want?

This is what it should be about ...

Your employees should be treated as you would have wanted to be treated when you were in school (and when you were an employee yourself at some point in your life). You should be able to paraphrase something like this to your employees: *"I plan to spend the semester teaching you the answers so when it comes time for your final review, everyone will get an 'A.' "*

In business, communicating performance objectives and giving people the final exam questions ahead of time are the perfect ways to ensure that everyone is headed in the right direction. Once goals are clear, leaders should wander around and "teach people the answers" so when they get to the final exam, they all get an "**A**."

Start moving in the right direction ...

Here is a list of things to try that may make you a better leader:

1. Red lights stop progress; green lights do the opposite.

 STOP ADMONISHING FOR EVERY LITTLE FAULT.

 START PRAISING FOR EVERY LITTLE ACHIEVEMENT!

2. If you observe your employees doing things right, even partially right, you need to provide praise to motivate continued progress.

3. When is the last time you said "**Thank you**" or "**Job well done**" to one of your employees? The key is to <u>make it a part of your daily habits – every day</u>. Make a list of your employees, put it on your desk in your office, and then put a checkmark next to each name when you have complimented or thanked them, at least <u>once every day – DO IT EVERY DAY</u>. Each individual may find your new appreciation and actions strange at first, but don't give up. Just wait and be persistent. YOU WILL SEE POSITIVE RESULTS!

Start catching people doing things right;
*then, <u>**PRAISE and REWARD**</u> the progress – any progress at all,*
*and I emphasize <u>**ANY PROGRESS AT ALL**</u>.*

Domination is unacceptable ...

Leadership is to be exercised.
But, domination is unacceptable.

Consider discarding your thought processes that go with a term like "management," and replace it with "leadership" or "coaching."

Management connotes the following images: referee, judge, mediator, manipulator, boss, critical analyst, etc. These descriptions can be seen as controlling.

Leadership, on the other hand, describes qualities such as trust, vision, guidance, imagination, mentorship, praise and direction. These are more acceptable and productive attributes.

The leadership paradox...

As a leader, you don't want your tombstone to read:
(paraphrased from Tom Peters)

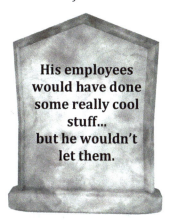

His employees
would have done
some really cool
stuff...
but he wouldn't
let them.

Superb business leaders epitomize paradoxes ...

1. They are tough and uncompromising about their value systems, BUT they care deeply about and respect their employees.
2. These exceptional leaders demand that each team player be an innovative contributor, BUT they are open in support of those people who dare to take risks and try something new as long as the leader's values are supported.
3. Great leaders must cultivate passion and trust, BUT at the same time, leaders must concentrate unmercifully on the details.

Unfortunately, <u>most leaders resolve the paradoxes by avoiding them</u>. You must confront the paradoxes, own them, live them and celebrate them if you want to make headway in achieving excellence.

Being a leader <u>is not</u> about ability.
Being a leader <u>is</u> about responsibility.

CHAPTER 3: WHAT'S REALLY IMPORTANT?

You're in the people business ...

Although the financial acumen outlined in this book is absolutely vital to your success, <u>you do not sell financial control; you sell a service to real people</u>. When did you ever hear that a great company (think Apple or Disney) was characterized by the remark: *"That company has a great budget."*

Since your business is in the people business, you must demand innovation from your people (i.e., <u>everyone</u> on your team – general office through clinical staff through office managers). Turn these people into super-sensitive detecting instruments for observing what customers really want and what new methods might be instituted or developed to achieve the customers' desires and the profitability of the practice.

> *Leaders don't try to transform employees.*
> *Leaders create opportunities for people*
> *and then encourage them to*
> *apply their talents to grasp those opportunities.*
> Tom Peters

All of these elements seem perfectly obvious, but again, the obvious does not always seem to perfectly associate with what you really do. Make an effort to carry out the obvious actions you need to be successful – i.e., **<u>DO WHATEVER IT TAKES</u>**.

> *It's a leader's job to make time today*
> *to ensure that there is a tomorrow.*
> Ken Blanchard

Listen, listen, and then, listen ...

> **Most people do not listen with the intent to understand.**
> **They listen with the intent to reply.**
> Stephen Covey

When it comes to relations with your employees, start by paying attention to your people -- really **LISTENING** to them. Then, **TAKE ACTION** on what you hear.

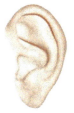

Consider this imaginary discussion between a doctor and another fellow doctor:

- Doctor #1: *"What's one of the toughest things in this business?"*
- Doctor #2: *"Listening to our employees."*
- Doctor #1: *"They just don't seem to understand what I'm trying to tell them."*
- Doctor #2: *"Yeah. That's why the listening part is so hard."*

> **Whenever a problem arises, the tendency is to try to talk**
> **your way out of it. But, sometimes you win by shutting up**
> **and listening your way out of it.**
> Thaler

What is wrong with the above dialogue? Anyone should be blinded by the obvious. Who should be doing the listening, the doctor or the employees? Unfortunately, the obvious must not be as obvious as one would assume. If it were, more owners would start listening to employees instead of dictating to them. By the way, the listening example above also applies to conversations between the doctor and the patient.

> When it comes to listening, you don't get what you demand, you get what you earn.

> **Leaders earn authority through**
> **listening, understanding and trust.**
> Klaus Balkenhol

CHAPTER 4: THE MUTUAL FUSSINESS FACTOR

"Mutual fussiness" occurs when employers and prospective employees both have high standards for what they will accept for hiring someone or for being hired.

1. **On the part of the employer**, artificially high standards often come in the form of unwillingness to train, low wages, weak benefits, etc.
2. **On the part of the prospective employee**, it's wages that are not high enough, not having the proper training, or having wages or salaries not as high as what they've had in the past.

In some cases, the skills gap is less explained by people who are not qualified and, at least partially, more explained by this mutual fussiness on the side of both prospective employees and employers.[7]

If employers want good people, they have to be willing to develop them.

1. Train those who have the right attitudes and abilities but not have the know how to take action themselves.
2. Pay what the market demands for good workers.
3. Provide benefits that retain good workers.

Employees, on the other hand, must recognize:

4. What got them hired may not get them promoted.
5. Skills must be updated through self-training.
6. Want to make more? Obviously, then <u>deliver more value</u>.

Unfortunately, many of the "artificial high standards" are based on a mentality of rewarding seniority versus ability where many people have twenty years of one year's worth of repeated experience.[8]

---

[7] Zellmer, Michael, PhD. Interview. 4/19/18.

[8] Smith, Mark S. A. Discussion. 4/23/18.

CHAPTER 5: WHEN STAFF MEMBERS RESIST

Despite your good intentions, measuring, monitoring, etc., there are a number of reasons why staff may resist:

- They think you don't trust them to do their job well.
- They want to be "empowered" and not "second-guessed."
- They don't want to disappoint you.
- They want full credit and don't want to share rewards.
- They take pride in not needing your attention.
- They are not interested in improving.
- They don't think your monitoring will add any value.[9]

*Employees today want a team relationship with you,
not a top-down hierarchy.
Listen to their suggestions,
then let them lead you to success.*

Dealing with these concerns up front will prepare employees to think like you think. When you obtain a mutual understanding and agreement on how the processes should occur, you will find that your monitoring will be a welcome support to making things happen. Anyone who depends upon others to get things done will "inspect what they expect" and do it in a way that makes it a positive experience for all the parties involved.

*You are the leader of your practice.
You are also the victim of the quality of your leadership.*
Mark S. A. Smith

---

[9] Partners in Leadership, July 2009.
https://www.partnersinleadership.com/insights-publications/inspect-what-you-expect

CHAPTER 6: EMPLOYEE HANDBOOKS

Although there are many laws requiring employers to notify employees of certain workplace rights, there are actually no federal or state laws specifically requiring an employer to have an employee handbook, and there are plenty of doctor/owners who choose *not* to have one. Creating and maintaining an employee handbook, however, shows good leadership.

A well-prepared employee handbook will answer many of the routine questions that would otherwise end up on the desk of the doctor/owner or office manager. So, when employees know to look in the handbook first, it saves management time.

An employee handbook is a useful tool for providing employees with the information that, by law, must already be delivered in writing (e.g., equal employment opportunity, EEO, statements).

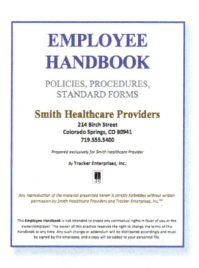

Rather than provide employees with a haphazard pile of mandatory written notices that show you are complying with the law and then attempting to document that those notices were received, it makes sense to collect them into an organized, easy-to-use handbook or similar document. It also makes sense to give the employees a source that discusses all they need to know about your practice. Finally, a legally compliant and up-to-date employee handbook may even provide legal protection if an employer's policies or practices are ever challenged in court.[10]

---

[10] BLR. Brentwood, TN. 2018. http://www.blr.com/About

What to include in an Employee Handbook

Before your employee handbook is written, you should take the time to determine what is important to you and your practice. Important issues can be things like the employee's ability to use cell phones at work, dealing with the appropriate way (or inappropriate way) that employees discuss the employer in chat rooms or on blogs after hours, etc. One of the most important things to remember is that your handbook needs to reflect the way you want to do business. If you write a policy, be prepared to enforce the policy -- whether it is a policy setting limits or a policy supporting goals. You need to have your handbook be a true reflection of how your practice operates.

Legal policies should include:

- Family medical leave policies
- Equal employment and non-discrimination policies
- Worker's compensation policies
- Accommodation for disabilities
- Military leave
- Maternity leave
- Breast-feeding accommodations

Disclaimers should include:

- **Handbook is not a contract**: It's important to point out that the handbook is just that, a handbook that explains how your practice works. It should never make any promises about continued employment.
- **Handbook trumps previous policy documents**: It should make clear that it is the ultimate word on company policies.
- **Subject to change**: The policies in the handbook may be subject to change at any time.
- **Acknowledgment page**: It should state that the employees understand it is their responsibility to read and follow the policies. The employees sign it (admitting that they have read it), return the original to you and then, the employees receive a copy of the acknowledgment page with their signature.

Other sections to include:

- **Practice History**. This discusses the practice and its mission.
- **Paid Time-Off Policy**. This spells out:
  - How vacation time is earned and paid
  - How the employee should schedule time off
  - Holidays observed, including how employees will be compensated for the holidays.
  - Sick leave, family medical leave, maternity leave and other types of leave, such as military and spousal leave.
- **Employee Behavior**. Discusses attendance, meal breaks, rest periods, general expectations of conduct, a policy against employee harassment, discrimination, smoking, substance abuse, how employees may use personal cell phones, the Internet or email, conflict resolution and a dress code.
- **Pay and Promotions**. This explains the practice's:
  - Methods of payment
  - How often and when are paydays and how many pay periods there are in a year
  - What the overtime policy is
  - Defines work hours
  - Discusses the pay grades
- **Benefits**. Includes benefits offered (e.g., medical, dental, vision, life insurance, etc.) and
  - Who is eligible
  - Full-time vs. part-time
  - When to enroll

> Although having an employment law attorney prepare the employee handbook is recommended, if you or someone else in your office prepares the employee handbook, make sure the document is approved by an attorney familiar with employment law.

Even though an employee handbook is not legally required, it is ABSOLUTELY needed and is necessary. It lets the employees know what your policies are, and it demonstrates proof that they have agreed to your policies. It also gives them a foundation for understanding their responsibilities, how they can advance, what benefits are available to them, etc., etc. **JUST DO IT**.

Sample of Employee Handbook Table of Contents
Table of Contents

Employee Orientation 5
    Welcome... 6
    Our Philosophy.. 7
    Our Mission.. 7
    Employee Characteristics... 8
    Purpose of Manual... 9
    Employer/Office Manager Directives 9
    Licensure... 9
    Legal Entitlement to Work in the USA 9
    Employee Training/Probationary Period 10
    Part-time and Full-time Employees 10
    Employee Orientation Checklist 11

Employee Attendance 12
    Attendance 13
    Office Hours 13
    Time Clock.. 13
    Rest Periods and Lunch Breaks 14
    Overtime 14

Employee Benefits.. 15
    Holidays 16
    Vacation Time 16
    Bonuses.. 17
    Well/Sick/Personal Time.. 17
    Extended Sick Time 18
    Office Closure.. 18
    Health Care Plan 18
    Dental Care Plan 18
    COBRA 19
    Worker's Compensation 19
    Continuing Education... 20
    Uniforms 20
    Emergency/Funeral Leave 21
    Maternity Leave 21
    Family and Medical Leave... 21
    Election Day 22
    Jury Duty 22
    Inclement Weather... 22

Employee Handbook Table of Contents

Employee Compensation.. 23
    Wage and Salary Administration 24
    Paydays 24
    Overtime 24
    Authorization to Make Payroll Deduction 25
    Total Compensation Worksheet 26
Employee Evaluation 27
    Performance Evaluation (Employer).. 28
    Performance Evaluation (Employee) 31

Position Descriptions... 33
    Owner, Dentist, Office Manager 34
    Office Manager, Billing Manager 35
    Receptionist, Office Manager 36
    Dental Hygienist.. 37
    Hygiene Coordinator/Assistant.. 38
    Metabolic Typing 38
    Dental Assistant 39
    Lab Technician 42
    Ordering Supplies.. 42
    Sterilization 43

Team Meetings 44
    Guidelines 45
    Team Meeting Minutes Form 46

Environmental Workplace.. 47
    General Information on Workplace Safety 48
    Blood-borne Pathogens Standards 49
        Exposure Control Plan 49
        Compliance Methods 49
        Uniform Maintenance 49
        Hepatitis B Vaccination.. 50
        Post-exposure Evaluation 50
    Hazard Communication Standard 50
        Hazard Communication Program 50
        Labeling 50
    X-ray Monitoring... 50
        Operator Protection 51
        Patient Protection 51
    Building Safety 51
        Evacuation 51
    Medical Emergencies 52

Employee Handbook Table of Contents

Office Protocol 52
    Cleanliness 52
      Noise 52
      Special Precautions 52
    Hepatitis-B Vaccine Consent (Form) 53
    Housekeeping Schedule 54
    Housekeeping Schedule 55
    Required Posters 55

Patient Contact 56
    Personal Appearance 57
      Cleanliness 57
      Uniform 57
      Hair and Nails 57
      Accessories 57
      Personal Habits 57
    Confidentiality 58
    Patient Communication 58
      Telephone Communication 58
      Treatment Communication 59
    HIPAA 59

Working Together 60
    Teamwork 61
    Human Relations 61
    Telephone Usage 62
      Ten-Step Phone Script 63
    Building Security 64
    Food 64
    Bulletin Board 64
    Housekeeping 64
    Harassment 65
    Disciplinary Process 65
      Major Violations of Rules of Conduct 66
      Minor Violations of Rules of Conduct 66
    Termination 67
    Resignation 67
    Exit Interviews 67
    Personnel Records 68
    Keep Us Informed 68
    Notification 68

Acceptance Letter 69
    Acknowledgement of Receipt (Form) 70

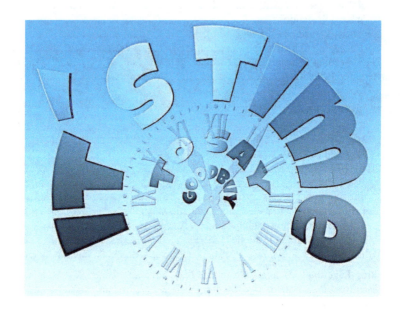

Letting go means coming to the realization that some people are a part of your history but not a part of your destiny.
Klaus Balkenhol

CHAPTER 7: WHEN IT'S TIME TO PART WAYS

When is it time to move on?

Hire and retain ONLY those with TOP TALENT.
No one else will do.
Talent does not just support your brand.
IT IS YOUR BRAND.

If you (the doctor/owner) are meeting the standards of being a great leader, <u>you must expect high standards from your employees</u>. If you have done all you can to train, monitor, measure and evaluate their performance and visit with them about that performance on a regular basis (be absolutely certain that you have documentation regarding these steps and provide the employee with a copy), and if they are not willing to comply, say "thank you" and "goodbye."

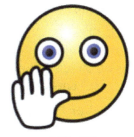

BYE, BYE

If all else fails, remember this statement from Tom Peters:

LIFE IS TOO SHORT.
Don't work with people who are dishonest,
who don't keep their word,
who only care about themselves,
and who are jerks.

Always remember, however, the old saying: "*What goes around, comes around.*" Let your employee go with dignity. Never hold a grudge. You never know when the two of you might need each other in the future. Besides, disgruntled employees can cause you pain in the future, e.g., legal considerations, Internet complaints, etc. Don't be afraid to simply say: "*It's not working out. We appear to have different goals. I wish you the best.*"

Do you need to give a reason for employee dismissal?

In the United States, employees generally can be released (i.e., fired) for good cause, bad cause, or no cause at all (at will). Employment in the United States typically is considered "at will," or terminable by either the employer or employee for any or no reason whatsoever. Legal exceptions to the rule seek to prevent wrongful terminations. You need to consider these exceptions before you let an employee go.

Employment-At-Will. Definition: A common-law rule that an employment contract of indefinite duration can be terminated by either the employer or the employee at any time for any reason (also known as terminable at will). [11]

The following exceptions address terminations that, although they technically comply with the employment-at-will requirements, are not deemed just or fair to employees.

1. **Public Policy Exception**: This prevents terminations for reasons that violate a State's public policy. It addresses the situation where an employee is wrongfully discharged when the termination is against an explicit, well-established State's public policy. For example, an employer cannot terminate an employee for filing a workers' compensation claim after being injured on the job or for refusing to break the law at the request of the employer. Seven states have rejected the public-policy exception: Alabama, Florida, Georgia, Louisiana, Nebraska, New York, and Rhode Island.
2. **Implied Contract Exception**: This prohibits terminations after an implied contract for employment has been established; such a contract can be created in the form of either oral assurances or expectations created by handbooks, policies, or other written assurances. Examples include employee handbook provisions that state that employees will be disciplined or terminated only for "just cause" or under other specified circumstances, or provisions that indicate that

---

[11] The Free Dictionary. Farlex. 2017.

an employer will follow specific procedures before disciplining or terminating an employee. Oral representations such as saying that employment will continue as long as the employee's performance is adequate also may create an implied contract that would prevent termination except for just cause. Employers can prevent written assurances from creating an implied contract by including a disclaimer characterizing those assurances as company policies that do not create contractual obligations. Employers should refrain from making any assurances to employment in the employee handbook. This exception is recognized in 38 states.

3. **Covenant of Good Faith**: Only six western states (Alaska, California, Idaho, Nevada, Utah, and Wyoming) have adopted this exception. The good-faith covenant has been interpreted to mean either that employer personnel decisions are subject to a "just cause" standard or that terminations made in bad faith or motivated by malice are prohibited.

Employers must be wary when they seek to end an employment relationship for good cause, bad cause, or, most importantly, no cause at all.[12]

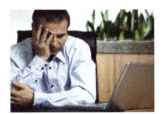

An in depth discussion on Leadership including preparation of an Employee Handbook is beyond the scope of this book. If you would like help preparing to be a great Leader, or if you would like help preparing an Employee Handbook, ask me about what we offer and how we can help you by emailing me at pjp@trackerenterprises.com.

---

[12] Charles J. Muhl. Former economist with The Bureau of Labor Statistics.

Leadership Summary:

1. Understanding the basic concepts of leadership
2. The ideal Performance Management Process
   a. Philosophy & Purpose
   b. Goal setting
   c. Educating and coaching
   d. Observing
   e. Monitoring and measuring progress
   f. Meeting and updating frequently
   g. Praising and redirecting at all steps along the way
3. Why listening is so important
4. The Mutual Fussiness Factor
   a. Employer
   b. Employee
5. What options do you have when staff members resist?
6. The importance of an Employee Handbook and what to include
   a. Legal policies
   b. Disclaimers
   c. All other items of importance
      i. Practice history and vision
      ii. Time-off policies
      iii. Employee behavior
      iv. Pay and promotions
      v. Benefits
      vi. Reasons for disciplinary action
      vii. Termination
      viii. Letter of Acknowledgement
7. Understanding "Employment at Will"
8. When and how to let an employee go

Leadership Action Plan: The Road Map

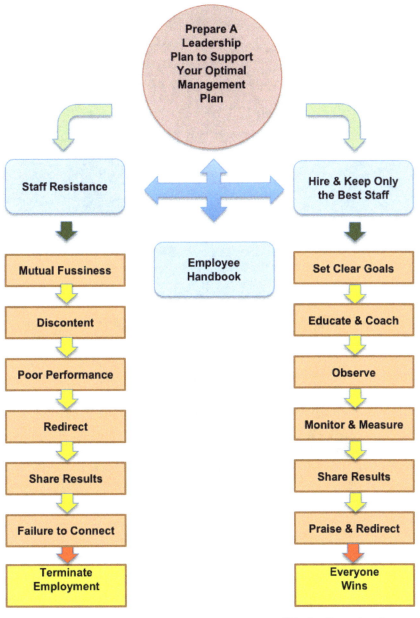

©Tracker Enterprises, Inc.

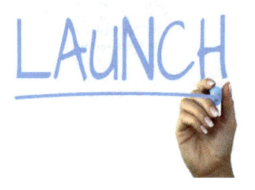

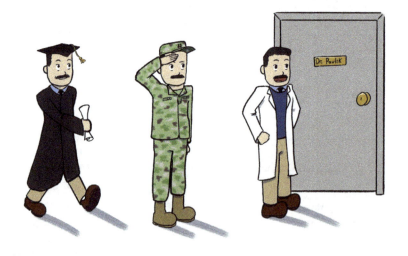

Section II: Launch

Chapter 8: My Story Begins With My Launch

Phase 1: The long preparation ...

The future looked great. Success was a given. I had just graduated with a healthcare doctoral degree (nine years of undergraduate, graduate, and post-graduate school to get my healthcare degree). I couldn't wait to give my new patients the care they deserved. My goals were to provide exceptional service and care. The byproduct of that service, in addition to making me feel good, was that my efforts would result in a nice cash flow. It seemed to be a given that my family and I would never want for life's essentials, along with the other amenities (plenty of respect and play money) that go along with being a doctor.

After graduating, I spent several fruitful years in the military. It was a great experience – work from 7:30 to 4:30, be on call once every two months, go to continuing education courses at the government's expense, and spend my non-patient treatment time watching and learning from great specialists. I gained the hands-on knowledge and experience to be a good healthcare provider.

Upon completing my military duty, I was ready to forge my own future by opening a family healthcare practice. I was fully aware that money was needed for equipment, rent, and operating capital (in the event things went a little slower than anticipated).

Phase 2: Spending time on the couch ...

After leaving the military, I frequently reclined on my living room sofa and stared at the vaulted ceiling in our small two-bedroom apartment, pondering whether leaving the military had been the right decision.

To give you a little background, several months earlier, I had turned in my resignation to the U.S. Army – a decision that was unexpected since I had planned on making a career in the military. This came about due to some unfortunate adjustments my colonel had made regarding my next assignment. The original plan included my wife to accompany me. The new plan ordered me to a 13-month assignment at the Korean DMZ without family. I opted to leave the military – a hard decision since, as I said, I had enjoyed the lifestyle and had learned so much about treatment options and dealing with a myriad of patient types and healthcare problems. Well, that part of my life was now over.

I made up my mind that deciding to enter private practice was the right thing to do – no associateship or corporate atmosphere for me; I wanted to be my own boss.

At first, my optimism was off the scale. I had been offered an opportunity to share office space with an established and well-respected doctor with no money down. Then, a week before I was supposed to start practicing, he told me that he had decided to give that opportunity to a recent graduate who was a friend of his family. I was devastated. That sofa meditation process began to repeat itself every afternoon – nowhere to go and no place to be.

When you have exhausted all possibilities, remember this:
You haven't.
Thomas Edison

Eventually, with luck, I managed to find another opportunity with two other established doctors. However, this time the circumstances were slightly different. Unlike the no-money down scenario with the previous offer, I was now obligated to put up a five-figure down payment that was to cover my "entrance fee" and the equipment necessary since the space I was offered was unfinished (i.e., unequipped and unfurnished).

To get started, I borrowed money from the banks and supply companies. Luckily, that process went easily for me.

I thought I knew everything I needed to start a practice. It would be easy. When I was seeing patients in the Army, I imagined what my charges would be for each patient, write down the dollar amounts, and calculate how much money would naturally come in when I was in private practice.

SIDE THOUGHT: Other doctor acquaintances, however, were not so lucky. Bankers wanted to see a financial statement (what was that?) with positive bottom lines. How was that possible; they hadn't even started their practices yet? In addition, bankers wanted a Business Plan (what was that?). The banks also wanted to use equity to secure the loans (these were doctors and success should be a given – who needs equity?). Many new doctors have no equity, so now what?

I had a nice clinical space to practice in. I was ready for the influx of eager patients. **REALITY CHECK – where were they?** The agreement that we three docs had was that we would rotate all new patients, the first going to Dr. 1, the second to Dr. 2, the third to me, (Dr. 3), UNLESS HOWEVER, the patients requested a specific doctor. Sounded fair at first BUT, patients

SIDE THOUGHT: I overlooked that unlimited amounts of patients were already a given in the Army and, unlike I was to later find out, the commanders made the soldiers show up for their appointments. Unfortunately, in private practice, I found that patients weren't as readily available and, once they were patients of record, they had no obligation to show up for their appointments and often did not.

had never heard of me. The other two docs were established and had a great reputation, so most new patients requested one of them, not me. I now had the opportunity to sit at my new desk in my new office and stair at the ceiling – a different location and a different view than I had on my home sofa, but the thoughts were no better than before. I started thinking how my doctoral education had ill-prepared me for the real life in the real business world that awaited me.

The Business Life Cycle Road Map

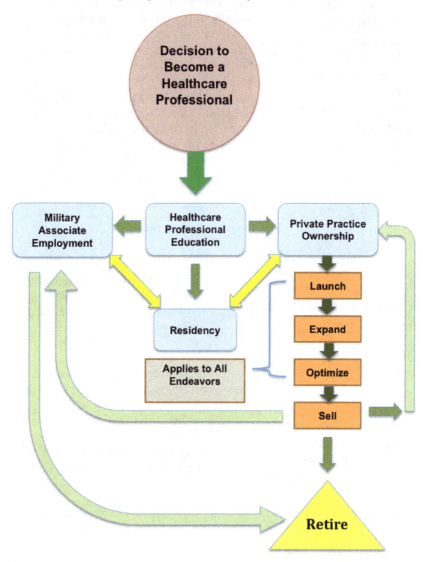

©Tracker Enterprises, Inc.

Chapter 9: How To Launch Your Career

You graduated – now what?

The first decision you must make is what to do after graduation.

- **Should you go into the military and once there, should you serve the minimum time required or make it a career?** My personal experience was very positive until near the end, as I said before. If you are facing some very heavy loan obligations from your education costs, the military can be very lucrative since pay starts immediately, bonuses to enlist are good, advanced degree programs are readily available and paid by the military, and the life-style can be very relaxing and social. The downsides include frequent relocation, reassignment often times without family, a corporate like atmosphere with the occasional bad boss, and a lower pay scale than what is typical in private practice. <u>FYI, most retired military healthcare professionals either go into practice themselves or work for someone else after the military. So, you should know what to do outside of the military anyway</u>.

- **Should you work for another owner?** This could include working as an associate for another healthcare provider(s) or working in a large corporate environment. Advantages include a fixed pay scale with vacation and benefits, specified hours, and reduced on-call schedules. Disadvantages include possibly not making as much money as you would if you were your own boss, your work schedule is not up to you, you take orders from someone else,

> EXAMPLE: A graduate may find an associateship program significantly more advantageous since, if you like to spend more time with your children, the associateship is definitely more flexible and less stressful. My experience has been that these providers seem to have the lifestyle that they desire more attainable when they are employees of someone else.

you may be doing procedures and/or seeing patients you don't like, and your contract may limit where you can practice in the future (see **Section VI** for more details).

- **Should you go into a specialty program?** The advantages are that you most likely will make a higher income than as a generalist. You will need to decide whether you are certain you can live with a limited treatment scope practice for the remainder of your career, whether you can afford the extra education, and whether you want to spend the additional time required in advanced training to become a specialist.

- **Should you become a private practice owner?** The advantages are that you are your own boss, you have the opportunity to set your hours, you do the procedures and see the patients you like, you take as much time off as you want, and you may have a larger personal income (provided you are willing to work for it) than in the other career options. The biggest downside is the responsibility – if you are not willing to work at seeing patients, being the most compassionate and caring provider in the marketplace, being a truly great leader, being available to deal with employee issues, and be willing to spend the time and effort to understand sound business essentials, then choose one of the other career options.

Eventually, you will have to understand business ...

- If you are planning on the military, whether you stay 2, 20, or 30 years, you will probably still decide to continue practicing in private or corporate practice after the military.
- If you go to work for another owner, you should understand what is being expected of you and why; you need to understand contracts, and you need to understand business so that you can negotiate for what you are worth.
- If you are going into a specialty program, you will, at some point, whether in two or six years, be going into private practice or going to work for someone else.
- If you are going into a practice as an owner, you MUST understand basic business principles to succeed.

CHAPTER 10: WILL YOU BE A SMALL BUSINESS?

Will your practice be considered a small business?

Healthcare professionals don't see their business as a small business. **It's a big business to them.**

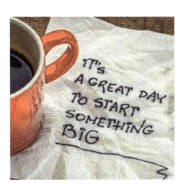

The SBA (Small Business Administration) defines a small business as an enterprise having fewer than 500 employees.[13] Unless you own or manage a large hospital, you are most likely considered to be a small business.

Why is your small business so important?

- They have generated over 65% of the new jobs since 1995.
- Over 50% of the working population works in small business.
- As of 2016, there were 28.8 million small businesses.[14]
- Every year 453,000 small businesses are started.
- These small businesses account for:
  - 99.7% of U.S. businesses
  - 49.2% of private-sector employment.
  - 42.9%of private-sector payroll.
  - 46% of private-sector output.
  - 43% of high-tech employment.
  - 98% of firms exporting goods.

If you don't seriously think your business and every business offering a product or service that benefits society is not important, think again. Unique and advantageous products and services give all of us a chance to improve our lifestyles. If your

---

[13] Nazar, Jason. Forbes/Entrepreneurs. September 9, 2013

[14] Bureau of Labor Statistics, www.sba.gov/advocacy/10871

practice offers a benefit to society (and you know it will since everyone needs healthcare), take every means possible to insure success. Give your financials the importance they deserve. Then, come up with a plan to prepare to meet and exceed your goals.

Challenges & Risks

> **Life is inherently risky.**
> **There is only one big risk**
> **you should avoid at all costs,**
> **and that is the risk of doing nothing.**
> Dennis Waitley

The following are census statistics that indicate the challenges and risks involved with the typical general small businesses:

- Only 50% will survive over 5 years.
- Only about one-third of those will survive 10 years or more.
- 82% of businesses fail because of cash flow problems.[15]

Why Do Practices Fail?

If you don't think that healthcare providers ever fail in business, think again. The most common reasons for practice failures are:

1. **Poor planning** – Doctors typically have a really hard time looking out a year or two in advance to plan where they want to be. The reason why is that they have been trained in the here and now looking at patients and fixing people. You absolutely must shift your brain to look out and plan for the future in a radically different way, and you probably need someone to help you to shift that thinking process and develop a plan. When you don't have proper planning, your business runs the risk of making decisions that seem good today but could have a negative long-term impact. You must include two types of planning:

---

[15] Bureau of Labor Statistics, BED; Update 2002- 2010, www.sba.gov/advocacy/7540/42371

a. Strategic Planning is the process of evaluating your business and decisions you face. The goal is to insure long-term success.
b. Operational (Tactical) Planning is the actions that must be taken according to the strategies you developed.

2. **Weak or inexperienced management** – You need to have the discipline to train yourself in understanding sound business concepts and how they apply to your practice.
3. **Inadequate financing** – To prepare for what you will need now and to prepare for what you will need in the future, you need to put yourself in a strong relationship with a banker.
4. **Poor location** – Don't buy a practice without understanding location sensitive issues.
5. **Increased competition** – Cutting your prices is no way to deal with competition. Solid marketing strategies are how you handle competition.
6. **Low sales or production** – If you aren't producing enough procedures and if the procedures are not valuable to the patients, your production will be low. Low production results in lower revenue; one follows the other (more later). You must concentrate on either high dollar production procedures or do a high volume of procedures.
7. **Not making changes when needed** – You must monitor what is happening everywhere in your practice, then measure what you monitored, then make adjustments to correct discrepancies, and then, start over again (more later). In today's business environment, the two most important questions affecting your business are "what if" and "what next." You need to be able to track your resources and expenditures until you can see every financial situation that could affect your business and then allow you the opportunity to make the smart adjustments necessary to prepare correctly for the future.

This is the first time in the history of business that you can be great at what you're doing today and be out of business tomorrow.
Ken Blanchard

53

The following representations may help you understand why other businesses fail. Do you see yourself in any of these?[16]

	Major Cause	Percentage of Failures	Specific Pitfalls
1	Incompetence	56%	Emotional Pricing Living too high for the business Nonpayment of taxes No knowledge of pricing Lack of planning No knowledge of financing No experience in record-keeping
2	Lack of Managerial Experience	33%	Poor credit Too rapid expansion Poor borrowing capacity
3	Lack of Supply & Product Experience	10%	Carry inadequate inventory No knowledge of suppliers Wasted marketing
4	Neglect, Fraud	1%	Poor management

Ten Leading Management Mistakes

1 Going into business for the wrong reasons
2 Bad advice from family and friends
3 Being in the wrong place at the wrong time
4 Entrepreneur gets worn out and/or underestimated the time requirements
5 Family pressure on time and money commitments
6 Pride
7 Lack of market awareness
8 Entrepreneur falls in love with the business
9 Lack of financial responsibility and awareness
10 Lack of a clear plan and focus

---

[16] Statistic Brain, https://www.statisticbrain.com/startup-failure-by-industry

CHAPTER 11: HOW TO START YOUR PRACTICE?

What about the money you will need?

Healthcare education can leave doctors with up to $500,000 of debt (that's before you buy or build a practice, pay for a place to live, etc.). More thoughts to consider: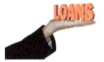

- "Hanging out a shingle" does not guarantee success; that's ancient thinking and can result in being ill prepared.
- Just being a good doctor is no longer enough. You must understand expenses (e.g., labor, supplies, facility, administration, and marketing) and cash flow.
- The biggest challenge is getting doctors to realize where and how their profits are leaking. On average, there's a 10% to 15% profit leak in a typical private practice. Much of that is tied to money owed to the practice by patients or insurers.[17],[18]
- They owe over $250,000 - $500,000 for their education.

Thirty years ago, a healthcare professional could go to any bank and borrow any amount of money necessary to fund a new practice. Lending institutions were comfortable that a doctor was a sure bet to be successful. Today, lending institutions have become more selective. My recent experience with healthcare professionals seeking to find the dollars to finance a start-up practice, to purchase an existing practice or to obtain financing for new equipment, etc. has proven more difficult. Although lenders are currently flush with cash, they have become very demanding. They are concerned with the huge increases in doctor to patient ratios, the significant and continuing growth of managed healthcare systems (HMOs, PPOs, etc.), the ever growing, mismanaged and increasing accounts receivables, and recent foreclosures and bankruptcies of doctors of all kinds.

---

[17] Ike Devji, J.D., Doctors Going Broke in the News> January 13, 2012

[18] http://chiro.org/wordpress/2012/01/doctors-going-broke

What's the approval rate for small business loans?

- The current SBA 7(a) loan is a great option. Low interest rates and long repayment terms are excellent, but lenders require excellent credit. The maximum loan amount is $5 million.
- In 2016, big banks approved only 24% of funding requests.
- Institutional lenders (which include savings banks and life insurance companies) approved 63%.
- Small banks approved 49%.
- Alternative lenders (e.g., Henry Schein, etc.) approved 58%.
- Credit unions approved 42%.[19]

What is the average time to get funding?

- For a short-term loan, funding is usually less than 10 days.
- For an SBA loan, it is more than a month and a half.

What type of healthcare service do you provide?

Number of healthcare professionals in the United States:

- Doctor of Medicine (MD)   870,312[20]
- Doctor of Osteopathy (DO)   81,115
- Doctor of Dentistry (DDS/DMD)   195,722[21]
- Doctor of Chiropractic (DC)   80,000[22]
- Physician Assistants (PA)   106,200
- Physical Therapists (PT)   239,800[23]

---

[19] Bureau of Labor Statistics.
https://www.bls.gov/bdm/entrepreneurship/bdm_chart3.htm

[20] Journal of Medical Regulation, 2017.
https://www.fsmb.org/Media/Default/PDF/Census/2016census.pdf

[21] Munson & Vujicic, ADA, 2016.
http://www.ada.org/~/media/ADA/Science%20and%20Research/HPI/Files/HPIBrief_061
6_1.pdf

[22] American Chiropractic Assoc. https://www.acatoday.org/Patients/Why-Choose-
Chiropractic/Key-Facts

More than $800 billion in healthcare costs are processed each year; income potential should be limited only by a desire to succeed! Unfortunately, revenue gets depleted by these statistics:

- Providers spend $7 billion annually submitting claims.
- The Healthcare System wastes up to 24 cents out of every dollar on administrative costs or $6 billion annually.
- The average healthcare provider has more than $150,000 in accounts receivables with 10-20% being over 90 days.
- Most healthcare facilities receive at least 70 to 75 % of their income from third-party payers (i.e., insurance).
- Costs continue to rise for labor, technology, and insurance.

What business structure should you choose?

During the business lifetime of your practice, you will either elect or restructure to one of the following business entities:

- **Pass-through entities** (e.g., S-Corporation, LLC or Limited Liability Corporation, Individual Proprietorship, or Partnership) - Most small businesses are "pass-through" entities, meaning that profits flow through to the business owner's personal tax return and are taxed as ordinary income.

- **C-Corporation** - The new tax code cuts the corporate tax rate from a maximum of 35% to 21% (this applies to C-corporations). Remember, however, that owners of C-corps also pay a second tax on profits distributed as dividends to its owners/stockholders. Historically, this has been the main reason why so many small business owners have opted for the one-time taxation advantage of the pass-through entities. [24]

Sole Proprietorship

S Corporation

Limited Liability Corporation

Partnership

C Corporation

---

[23] Bureau of Labor Statistics. https://www.bls.gov/ooh/healthcare/physical-therapists.htm

[24] Simon, Ruth. *The Wall Street Journal*. February 23, 2018.

The majority of small businesses are S-corporations (42%) followed by LLCs (23%).[25]

You need to be able to answer the following questions first:

- "Will changing my practice structure cut my tax bills?"
- "Should I operate as a C-corporation, which pays its own taxes to the IRS, or as a pass-through company which pays taxes through the individual returns of its owner?"[26]

How to start the planning process ...

Successful small business owners typically start with an operational business plan (a system based on how your particular business operates, takes in income, and pays out expenses each month) that will offer the best chance for success.

The **average healthcare professional** does not prepare an operational business plan. It is essential that you begin to operate your practice as a proper business should operate.

> SIDE THOUGHT: A "plan" is a written account of an intended future course of action aimed at achieving specific goals.
>
> A "system" is defined as a set of things, actions, ideas and information that interact with each other and in so doing, alter and improve the functioning of other systems. It is an organized method, or set of procedures, that results in a condition of harmonious and orderly interaction.

Do you need a business plan?

A **Business Plan** is a document that summarizes the operational and financial objectives of a business and contains the detailed plans and budgets showing how the objectives are to be realized. It is the road map for the success of a business.

---

[25] Ruger, Michael. Greenbush Financial Group, LLC. 2018.

[26] Mercado, Darla. Your Money Your Future. CNBC. January 9, 2018

For anyone starting a business, **it's an essential first step**. If startup financing is anticipated, a Business Plan may be required by the lending institutions. You must have a Business Plan that demonstrates how the proposed practice will be profitable.

Because the Business Plan contains detailed financial projections about your practice's future performance, it's an incredibly useful tool both for start-up practices and for everyday business planning and, as such, should be reviewed regularly and updated as required. Your Business Plan should provide information on calculating your start up and operating expenses and should include a budget to back it up.

You can have a great idea for a business and excellent operational plans but, if the Business Plan demonstrates that you may not make enough income after expenses to be profitable, then the business model is not viable. If the plan doesn't look like it will work, go back and redo it until it does.

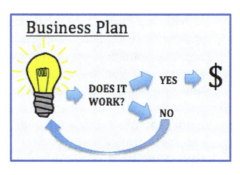

A typical Business Plan will include:

1. Executive Summary
2. Industry Overview
3. Market Analysis
4. Competitive Analysis
5. Marketing Plan
6. Management Plan
7. Operating Plan
8. Financial Plan
9. Appendices and Exhibits

A more detailed explanation of the above components follows:

1. **Executive Summary** - Summarizes the key elements of the business plan and is the first thing anyone looking at your plan reads so it is critical that your summary is outstanding.
2. **The Industry** - Overview of the healthcare sector your business will be a part of including industry trends.
3. **Market Analysis** - An examination of the target market for your healthcare services including location, demographics, target market, and how that market is currently serviced.
4. **Competitive Analysis** - You need to distinguish your business from the competition, persuading the reader of your plan that your business will be able to compete.
5. **Marketing Plan** - A detailed explanation of your sales strategy, pricing plan, proposed advertising and promotion activities, and product or service benefits. This is where you present how you're going to get your services to market and how you're going to persuade people to buy them.
6. **Management Plan** - An outline of your practice's legal and management structure including your management team, external management resources and human resources needs.
7. **Operating Plan** - Description of your practice's location, facilities, equipment, employees needed, inventory suppliers and requirements, and any other applicable operating details, such as a description of the healthcare service process.
8. **Financial Plan** - Description of funding requirements and detailed financial statements. This is where you will present the three main financial documents of any business: balance sheet, income statement and cash flow projections.
9. **Appendices and Exhibits** - At the end of your plan, include any additional information that will help establish the credibility of your business plan such as marketing studies, photographs of your products and services, and contracts or other legal agreements pertinent to your business.[27]

---

[27] Ward, Susan. *The Balance*, https://www.thebalance.com/business-plan-outline-2947032

The days of "hanging out a shingle"
with a small amount of funding,
even less planning,
and having patients stumble in your door
are gone forever!

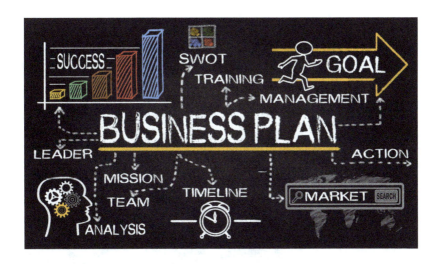

Choose the advisor who best matches your identity.

And remember,

If they don't have the scars, they don't have the wisdom.
Mark Smith

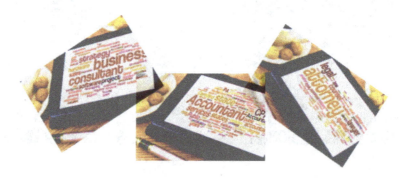

Your advisory staff and what you should expect?

With all of your advisors (e.g., certified public accountants, bookkeepers, financial advisors, healthcare consultants and attorneys, obviously all assumed to be looking out for your best interests), it is my experience that doctors who desire to understand their businesses better tend to encounter resistance from their advisors. 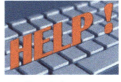 These advisors want to have you do it their way; they tend to discourage your involvement in understanding the business side of your practice. After all, you're a doctor, not a business expert – i.e., stay where you belong! These are your advisors, however, and you need to continue listening to them. If they do claim to provide 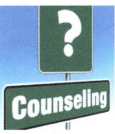 everything you need, however, why do so many practices barely get by? So, start taking control of your business. If they don't like it, find someone else.

You may be thinking that you can outsource interpretations of all of the financial and operational information. While I am completely committed to outsourcing anything that others can do to free up my time, I am also a firm 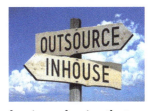 believer that you need to understand some business basics that specifically apply to your practice. In addition, I suggest that you do not take advice from someone new to or not familiar with your particular healthcare industry. Work with someone who has "walked the walk."

An in depth explanation of how to prepare a Business Plan and more comprehensive information on this section is beyond the scope of this book. If you would like notifications about training programs we provide on these subjects, ask me about what we offer and how we can help you by emailing me at pjp@trackerenterprises.com.

SECTION II: SUMMARY & LAUNCH ACTION PLAN

Launch Summary:

1. Where are you now?
   a. Healthcare student
   b. Residency program
   c. Healthcare faculty
   d. Hospital staff
   e. Military
   f. Associate (employee)
   g. Practice owner
   h. Healthcare Service Organization employee
   i. Looking at retiring or transitioning
2. Which of the following stages of your Business Life Cycle are you experiencing or preparing to enter?
   a. Launch
   b. Expand
   c. Optimize
   d. Sell
3. How well do you understand basic business principles?
4. What should you avoid to prevent failure?
   a. Poor planning
   b. Poor management
   c. Inadequate financing
   d. Poor location
   e. Increase competition
   f. Low production
   g. Not adapting to change
5. Obtaining sources of financing
6. Choosing the correct business structure
   a. Sole Proprietor
   b. S-Corp
   c. C-Corp
   d. LLC
7. Advisory Team: Choose an accountant, attorney and other advisors who are experienced in your field of healthcare.

Launch Action Plan: The Road Map

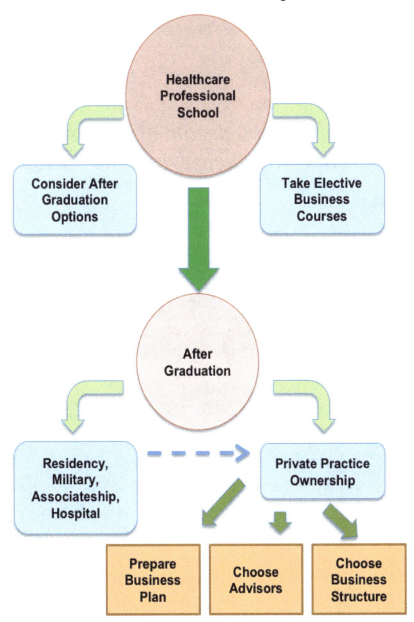

©Tracker Enterprises, Inc.

Those who dream of success dream with their eyes wide open.

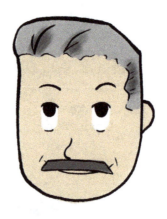

Section III: Expand

Chapter 12: My Story Continues - Expanding

After three years of struggling, my patient load was at a point where my free time in between patients was gone - forever. Revenue was coming in at a clip that was supporting my overhead and my family, to purchase a home, to get new cars and to purchase the toys I wanted. I didn't have the need to question my abilities to pay off new debt. Since the revenue stream seemed to be unlimited, my purchases of new equipment continued to increase – I wanted the best. I was making money in spite of my inabilities to understand business.

My business acumen was at best, elementary, so my financial decisions were based more on emotion and wants, not on needs or on a solid financial system.

If I went to the annual healthcare convention and saw something that would help my patients and make treatment easier or better for me, I bought it. If I wanted a new car for my family or for my recreational needs, I bought it. If I wanted a new house, I bought it.

In my defense, I did base my purchasing decisions loosely on a financial statement called a Profit and Loss Statement (or P&L) that I received every month from my accountant (I was smart enough to have an accountant even in the early stages of my career). Here's the way I saw it: if the bottom line on the P&L showed a black number that didn't have a minus sign in front of it or wasn't in parentheses, I started dreaming of a new item to purchase. If the statements were "in the black" for three months in a row, I felt I had carte blanche to do what I wanted. How's that for business acumen?

Fate was a harsh master. My timing for purchases was not always ideal, however. It seemed that just after I had supplicated myself to a new financial obligation, the next few months showed that my P&L bottom lines were not "in the black." In addition, for some reason unknown to me, even in my good months, I was being challenged to meet my loan obligations. I met with my accountant who told me that I should have also been looking at a financial statement called the Balance Sheet. No one told me that.

Well, I found out that the Balance Sheet showed a few slightly important items that were not on the P&L. The Balance Sheet showed both my practice's Assets (money in checking/savings that was useable and values regarding depreciation, equipment and goodwill that was not available as cash) and the Liabilities & Equity. The Equity demonstrated the distributions made to me, retained earnings, net income, etc.; this looked good on paper but realistically had no cash value. The Liabilities section, however, was the section that I had completely overlooked. It listed down payment loans on the practice, equipment loans, other practice loans, etc. that I was obligated to make payments on each month. This stuff did not show up on the P&L so I forgot about those payments that someone else (office manager, spouse, etc.) had been taking care of while I was in the clinic seeing patients. I was successful in spite of myself, but I now realized that I had to make some changes to cover all the expenses, and I did, including:

1. Paying attention to all expenses, not just the ones on the P&L.
2. Learning what information is in my financial statements.
3. Making more revenue including:
    a. Working more hours to increase production.
    b. Joining alternative insurances (PPOs, HMO, etc.).
    c. Hiring doctors to help with increased patient load.
    d. Hiring more staff to handle the increased load.
    e. Increasing my physical space requirement to handle the increased load at an increased rent payment.
    f. Opening a second office location.
    g. Buying more equipment and supplies for the above.
4. Becoming more of an innovative entrepreneur, a more responsible owner and manager, and a harder worker in the clinical setting.

CHAPTER 13: YOUR STORY CONTINUES - EXPANDING

A little more persistence, a little more effort,
and what seemed as hopeless failure
may turn to glorious success.
Elbert Hubbard

Does a healthcare degree guarantee success?

Don't assume that your scientific knowledge and clinical experience will automatically translate into the financial acumen needed to run your business – *it will not*. The ability to provide a health service *does not automatically qualify you to be an expert* on understanding the financial ins and outs of running a business.

There's no guarantee of financial freedom.
What you do dictates the outcome.
Kai Said

Are you immune to understanding business?

With all the education you received, you would assume you should be a sure bet for success. Unfortunately, unlike other businesses where customers pay for services and products at the time of sale, healthcare professionals have allowed themselves to accept and endure long delays between the time of service and the time when it is ultimately paid. These delays, coupled with a bureaucratic and cumbersome third-party billing structure, has resulted in diminishing cash flows.

Poor business acumen and volume of health claims has left many providers waiting (90 days or more) for reimbursement from insurers, slow-paying, or worse, non-paying patients, tort reform complications, Medicare, and Medicaid, etc. Since most healthcare providers receive <u>at least</u> 70-75% percent of their revenue from third-party payers, they need a strong understanding of their finances to survive these delays in compensation.

When operating a healthcare practice,
you are often caught in a paradox.

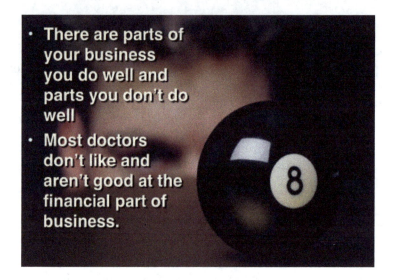

- There are parts of your business you do well and parts you don't do well
- Most doctors don't like and aren't good at the financial part of business.

The difference between the success and failure
of your practice may depend on
how you handle the parts of your business
that you do not do so well.

Do you need to have a business background?

Most healthcare professionals are visionaries (more on visionaries and entrepreneurs later) and experts in providing healthcare services. They are not trained to understand the financial part of their business and they do not like to spend the time analyzing their financials; so, they are not good at it. They delegate the finances to their bookkeeper, accountant, office manager, and/or financial advisor and then, if they take the time to do it at all, the 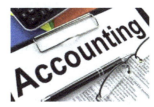 owner/doctors review reports that they may not understand.

How do you rank yourself?

On a scale of one to ten, with ten being outstanding and very successful, how do you rank yourself on knowing exactly how well your practice is doing financially and how well your business might adapt to changes, anticipated or not?

> *If you are not at a ten,*
> *what are you going to do about it?*
> *If you are at a ten, why not strive for an eleven?*

Do you need to understand financial statements?

If you're like most doctors or other healthcare professionals, you already spend 100% of your time with all of the things that you have to do to run your business - you have to stay on the cutting edge, stay ahead of the competition, serve your patients well, and be responsible for the cash. In addition to all of the above, and most importantly, you are expected to understand exactly what's going on financially with your practice.

> *Do you understand exactly*
> *what is going on with your business?*
> *If not, what are you going to do to correct it?*

Where do you want to go with your business?

You need to plan ahead. No matter how complete your current financial strategies are, you will, most likely, need to make some changes along the way. When things don't go exactly as planned, you will need alternative plans to help you make corrections to get you back on track toward meeting or exceeding your goals.

You need to be able to gain a better understanding of how you can accurately predict and react to the opportunities and consequences of changes, anticipated or not, so that you can make intelligent business decisions and increase profits. If you adhere to the firm financial rules that govern any good business, this will help you reach your goals.

> ***Are you going through financial changes,***
> ***anticipated or not?***
> ***How do you feel about that?***

Can you guarantee success?

> **You must be able to see the forest from the trees.**

Making guarantees to patients about the future of their health is usually not a good idea and would not be based on reality. Similarly, making guarantees in business is, at best, questionable. There will be, however, a few guarantees you can count on for your business:

- Your practice **will definitely deviate** from your original plan.

- Your practice **will continue to change** over the years.

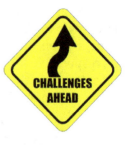

- At some point, **you will leave** your profession.

To successfully make the necessary adjustments in response to these deviations and changes, you must keep your practice business plan current.

Consider these questions:

- Is the business developing according to plan?
- If not, what adjustments do you need to make?
- Where do you want your business to be one year, three years, etc. from now, and how should you make the changes necessary to get you back on track?

Although creating an operational plan may seem like a *one-time* event, keeping it up to date and redirecting it as changes occur must be an *ongoing* task. This is achieved by constantly *asking yourself questions* about the state of your business and then, *updating your financial outlook*. This update can be done by doing *forecasting* and *what if scenarios*, ideally at a rate of once per month.

> You *must have the ability* to dissect the financial aspects of your company *at least once per month*.

Right now, you are probably making excuses ...

- My practice is different from everyone else's.
- If I offer a good product/service, I will be successful.
- Plenty of healthcare practices have been started and have done well and continue to do quite well without solid business tools.

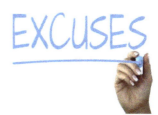

Think about what you need to do to arrive at a more successful outcome. Doctors have become complacent about accepting responsibility for their practices. In today's business climate, simply being a healthcare practitioner does not guarantee success.

It's time for you to break away from the "ordinary" way of looking at your business and EXPERIENCE a new way of preparing for success.

Thinking it through ...

Regardless of the type of existing healthcare model you own or want to own, you must be familiar with understanding financial statements. Once you have had the opportunity to evaluate the financial statements, you need to consider doing forecasting to make accurate predictions so that you can better plan to reach the goals you have set. If you are the average doctor or potential practice buyer, you lack some of the expertise necessary to make educated financial decisions. Consider using these experts: tax advisors, attorneys, transition experts, and small business consultants (especially those trained in operational management including budget, forecasting, and "what if" scenarios).

> *You*, the owner, will ultimately determine the fate of your business venture.

Most importantly, remember that all expenses are paid and all profits come out of revenue (and most revenue comes out of production). If you do not know how much revenue you need in order to accomplish your goals, how can you possibly know whether your business will be able to reach those goals or worse, whether you will be able to stay in business? So, how much money will you need to accomplish your goals? Is your practice generating the revenue needed? If not, you need to make adjustments.

Build the roadmap, follow it, and then learn to adjust if the path becomes blocked or if you see better ways to get to your destination. Without a clear direction or roadmap, how can you possibly know how to proceed?

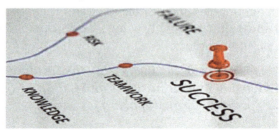

Know your 3 Ws:

- **W**here you are
- **W**here you've been
- **W**here you're going

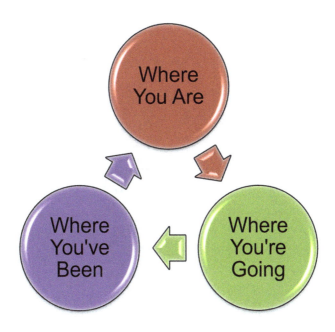

©Tracker Enterprises, Inc. 2018

Never ever make business decisions based on emotional whim or guesswork.

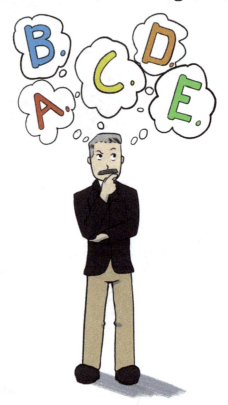

Listening to your gut should be a key in helping in decision-making, but analyze, analyze, analyze before leaping.

CHAPTER 14: THE GENESIS OF YOUR PRACTICE

What is your job description?

Every healthcare provider should start a practice with the hope of becoming an expert in three different jobs at the same time:

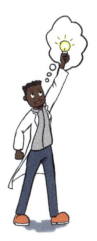

1. An Entrepreneur,
2. A Manager (a.k.a., Owner and CEO), and
3. A Technician.[28]

The **Entrepreneur** in you is the visionary or the dreamer. <u>You see an opportunity or need, and you invent a new or better way to satisfy it</u>. You see success as a given since you conceived it. This is one of the prime drivers in a doctor's interest in continuing education. (Side note:

Entrepreneur

why would you want to pay to learn new techniques and pay big bucks for new equipment when you have yet to utilize all of what you have learned and bought at previous courses?)

The **Manager** in you hopes to make order out of everything so that your practice can run smoothly. Ideally, you will have the time and ability to plan, lead, organize, and control all of the functions to keep the practice going. The Manager lives in the present, but needs to look into the future. You know that to succeed, you must understand your financial "numbers," boring and tedious as they may seem. The owner/executive in you typically thinks you can successfully manage your financials even though your knowledge and experience are usually concentrated in the service of healthcare. (How many of you have received formal training in financial management?)

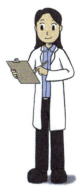

Manager/Owner

---

[28] Gerber, Michael E. The E-Myth. HarperCollins Publishers, Inc., 1995.

The **Technician** in you believes you know how to deliver the service. Because you believe you have the expertise to provide the best healthcare service in the marketplace, you are confident. <u>You are happiest working "on the assembly line" or "in the trenches," as I like to call it, since practice production comes primarily from the treatment you provide to your patients</u>.

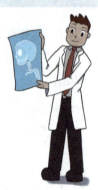

Technician

During the infancy of your practice, because customer demand is usually weakest at that time, the owner typically has no problem taking on the responsibilities of Entrepreneur, Manager, and Technician. You are starting a new business that, in your heart, you know will succeed. You are confident that the services you provide will be the best in the marketplace; you assume your intelligence will handle the Manager responsibilities (usually a doctor's weakest link). Regardless of your shortfalls, you are sure more new ideas will enter your Entrepreneurial mind when the need arises.

It is critical to have all three of these positions working at maximum efficiency for any business to succeed.

Growing pains ...

A typical successful, non-healthcare, small business owner spends 85% of the time as a Manager and no more than 5% of the time to devoted technical tasks. The Owner is fortunate to devote 10% of the time to being an Entrepreneur. Remember, these statistics apply to a successful non-healthcare general business. A healthcare provider, however, has nowhere near this time to devote to managerial duties. Usually, the Technician part consumes at least 90% of the time. Consequently, other business experts commonly conclude: *"Doctors make up the worst business owners and managers in the business marketplace."*

Vision without execution is hallucination.
Walter Isaacson

Examples of Time Spent in Successful vs. Healthcare Practice

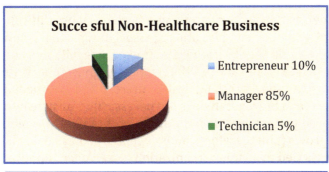

Succe sful Non-Healthcare Business

- Entrepreneur 10%
- Manager 85%
- Technician 5%

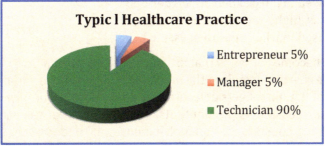

Typic l Healthcare Practice

- Entrepreneur 5%
- Manager 5%
- Technician 90%

Without a Technician, the services would never be produced properly. The services must be produced with great expertise and care; this is usually not a problem since the doctor has the needed training and clinical expertise. Without a Manager, however, there can be no way of controlling the business. Without an Entrepreneur, unfortunately, there can never be any innovation. Since little time and effort is allotted for the management and innovations needed to stay ahead of the competition and to managing finances, this unbalanced distribution of work can lead to less than ideal results.

As patient population increases and procedure demand increases, it will only be a matter of time before one or more of the other positions begin to lose their level of importance because of the overwhelming need to satisfy the patients' demands (for the Technician). You are forced to work harder, and longer hours force you to juggle all three responsibilities. After all, you must concentrate on the service because that's where you have your expertise. Unfortunately, if you do not also pay attention to the Owner/Manager position, you will lose sight of your finances.

Now, as the business grows and becomes more difficult to control, you decide to hire others (associates, partners, new staff, etc.) to pick up the slack where your expertise falls short or to help provide more services. Unfortunately, given time, since no one else has your foresight, desire, interest, and judgment, you realize that a bigger staff does *not* necessarily translate into an improved patient experience or more profitability. As your labor team grows (and therefore, labor expenses grow), so do all other expenses tied to a larger organization (e.g., higher supply costs, increased facility expenses, bigger debt services, higher administrative costs, increased marketing expenses, etc.).

It becomes obvious that as your business grows, you lose the ability to control it. Control gets delegated to other professionals (accountants, attorneys, consultants – all high expense experts) who not only take away some of your decision-making processes but also do not share your vision.

> If you do not focus on the product or service, quality and quantity will suffer resulting in decreased revenue and customer satisfaction.

The point of no return ...

Because you must continue to focus on the production (Technician) end of your business (that's what's bringing the money in, right?), managing shrinks in importance. Since you have delegated much of the financial responsibilities to outsiders, you lose contact with reality. Making good and well-thought-out business decisions now become almost impossible. Managing your practice's finances now becomes a nuisance since production has become your primary goal.

Without any warning, you may find yourself unable to make the practice and equipment loan payments, the huge staff salaries, and the practice facility expenses. That ever-so-helpful accountant that never indicated you had a problem now tells you that the only way out is to restructure or file for bankruptcy. (*Despite my business acumen early in my career, fortunately, I never experienced this but some other healthcare providers have.*)

There is another way ...

Your job, as the Owner/Manager, should be to *anticipate* the future. You must educate yourself so that all three of your job titles, Entrepreneur, Manager, and Technician, know exactly what to do and when to do it.

> ### Executives always see the big picture and yet appreciate the fine details.
> Mark S. A. Smith

To move in a positive direction, you need to formulate an operational business plan. It has to be written so that everyone (your staff, advisors, bankers, etc.) can understand your vision, be guided along the path toward mutual goals, and be given a plan (road map) to adjust back to the correct path when the way is temporarily lost. As healthcare providers, we know one thing without question:

> ### We understand that if we want to solve the problem, we have to get the right diagnosis.

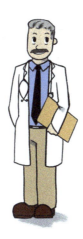

You have to understand accounting.
It's the language of business.
Unless you are willing to put in
the effort to learn how to interpret
financial statements,
you really shouldn't be in business.

Warren Buffett

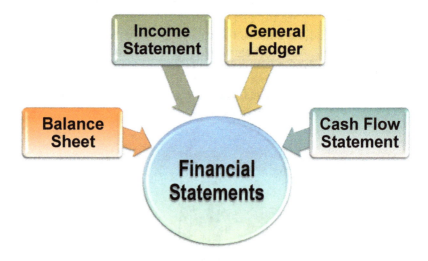

Chapter 15: Understanding Financial Reports

First, do you speak the language?

Production describes the amount or value you charge for the services and products you provide.[29] As all healthcare professionals have experienced, the amount charged is not necessarily the amount collected. Because of bad patient debts, insurance adjustments, etc., you rarely can depend on Production as a benchmark of what will end up in the bank.[30] *In the healthcare industry, this is what you provide for your patients and how much that service is really valued at.*

Revenue is the amount of cash generated by the sale of products or services associated with the practice's operations. In other words, revenue refers to all of the money (cash, checks, electronic credits, etc.) a practice takes in from doing what it does.[31] *This is the amount of cash, patient and insurance checks, credit card payments, etc. that your practice receives.*

Expenses are the costs to run a business and pay any debt due; i.e., the cost incurred in an organization's efforts to generate revenue, or the cost of doing business. [32] *For your practice, expenses may be in the form of actual cash payments (such as wages/salaries, clerical, clinical, lab expenses, diagnostic tests, facility, administrative expenses, etc.), depreciation of an asset, or an amount taken out of earnings (such as bad debts).*

> SIDE THOUGHT: Even though expenses are usually not considered to be profit-making activities, _expenses should always generate revenue_. If they don't, why do you have them? *Eliminate the waste.*

---

[29] Wikipedia. https://en.wikipedia.org/wiki/Production_(economics)

[30] Tyson, Eric. Small Business for Dummies. Wiley Publishing, 2003.

[31] Business Dictionary. www.businessdictionary.com/definition/revenue.html

[32] Business Dictionary. http://www.businessdictionary.com/definition/expense.html

Income, also referred to as **Net Income or Net Profit**, is the amount of cash that remains from the amount of revenue after accounting for all operating expenses.[33] *In addition to the above, subtract out any debt service noted on the Balance Sheet such as practice loans, equipment loans, school loans, etc.*

Profit is the financial benefit realized when the amount of revenue gained exceeds the expenses, costs and taxes needed to sustain the activity. Profit goes to the owners, who may or may not decide to spend it on the business.[34] *Doctors often take this profit as a year-end bonus or as dollars applied to new technology, etc., for the practice.*

Cash Flow describes the movement of money (cash, checks, electronic debits and credits) in and out of the business.[35] *It is the money the practice generates before repaying debt obligations.* It differs from Net Income in that it eliminates non-cash items such as depreciation, amortization and accounts receivable.

> *Owners drive* the business of their businesses, but *cash fuels* the engine.

The simplest way to imagine the importance of cash flow is to think of the balance in your checking account. Will that balance be enough to pay your bills when they come due? It is a fact that the further out you can predict your bank balance, the further out you can see problems and the longer you have to prepare.

In order to pay bills, you need to manage the money (revenue) coming in and the cash (expenses) going out, i.e., your *cash flow*. Therefore, the following formula works to keep you in business *only* if revenue *exceeds* expenses.

> **Cash Flow = Revenue (cash in) – Expenses (cash out)**

---

[33] Investopedia. https://www.investopedia.com/ask/answers/122214/what-difference-between-revenue-and-income.asp

[34] Investopedia. https://www.investopedia.com/terms/p/profit.asp

[35] Investopedia. https://www.investopedia.com/terms/c/cashflow.asp

There are a couple of ways to manage Cash Flow: (1) prevention (e.g., managing in such a way that you can foresee problems and can deal with them early on) and (2) cure (e.g., dealing with problems after they surface). Would you prefer catching strep throat, taking antibiotics and supplements and staying home to recover, OR would you rather prevent strep throat by avoiding exposure to others that have it and taking precautions to build up your immune system? Prevention is by far the best option.

If you have worked on prevention but still discover unexpected problems, you may face some painful choices:

1. **Borrow** from personal funds: not ideal, but it may be necessary.
2. **Delay paying vendors**: They depend on your payments to keep their own businesses afloat so that is not recommended.
3. **Delay payroll** – NEVER acceptable.
4. **Convince your patients to pay** their bills early – patients rarely want to pay for services in advance before seeing how much insurance pays. You need to change this philosophy, but that is a subject for another discussion.

> If your Expenses don't generate Revenue, why do you allow wasteful expenses in your business?

A much better solution is to have a close relationship with your banker. You do this by sending your bankers, especially those you have loans with and those you have an LOC (Line of Credit) with, current (quarterly and annual) financial reports along with forecasting reports, if available. This shows the bankers that you really have a handle on the financial health of your business. The more a banker knows about your business and, more importantly, the more he thinks you know about your business, the more confidence he will have in you, and the more willing he will be to help out if you get in a cash crunch. (This is why having an LOC available is always a good idea. Ideally, the best time to look into this is when your business is flush with cash, not when you are desperately in need of the money.)

The bottom line with cash flow management is to develop the tools and discipline to manage it consistently, to look for problems as far into the future as possible, and to set up a good plan for dealing with the problems you cannot avoid if they occur.

It is also important to understand that the profits indicated in your financial statements include more than just cash. For example, the cash may have been shifted, at some point in time, to other assets including such "non-liquid" assets" as inventory, accounts receivable, equipment, and/or real estate. You need real "cash on hand" to pay expected and unexpected expenses.

> Cash is the only true "liquid" asset.

Always keep in mind that your practice's bank account is the measure of your ability to pay bills, not what you have in non-liquid assets. For example, will you have the cash needed for payroll, will you have money to pay the rent, utilities, taxes, and supplies, debt service, and will you have money to pay for unexpected expenses? This is why you need to know how to project the following:

- Your future production
- Collect money due (accounts receivable)
- Remaining costs of doing business
- Dollars due for upcoming payrolls including payroll taxes and benefits.

> You absolutely must be able to *accurately predict* tomorrow's cash flow.

Since it is inevitable most businesses will have cash flow problems, you need to have contingency plans to get cash should your forecast show a shortage.

The ability to sort through the numbers, recalculate every upcoming months' projections, and analyze the results can be cumbersome, time-consuming, and dangerous if the right person is not doing the forecasting, spreadsheets, reports, analyses, and charts. If you need help, email me at pjp@trackerenterprises.com.

Second, do you understand the script

If the map doesn't agree with the ground, the map is wrong![36]

You don't need to memorize or understand all of the intricacies of the financial statements but, as an owner, the worst thing you can do, when presented with your practice's reports, is to *not ask questions*, or even worse, *not pay any attention* to the information provided. You must understand what stories the financials are telling you. You must know how the financial details affect your bottom line, in other words, the Profit or Net Cash Flow. This chapter is meant to get you to ask the right questions and then interpret the answers.

You need to be provided with certain reports that will help you understand the status of your business. Four different financial statements are typically prepared by accountants for businesses on a regular basis (e.g., monthly, quarterly, annually, etc.). These reports include the **Income Statement**, the **Balance Sheet**, the **General Ledger** and the **Statement of Cash Flows**.

> In order to stay in business, you must create a profit.

Income Statements

The **Income Statement** (also known as a Profit & Loss Statement or P&L, the Operating Statement, the Earnings Statement, the Statement of Operating Results, or the Statement of Earnings) summarizes your estimated revenue and expenses over a specified period of time (e.g., monthly, quarterly, and/or annually).[37] It shows all of the money a business earned (revenues) and all of the money a

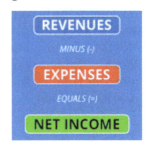

---

[36] Livingston, Gordon. *Too Soon Old, Too Late Smart*, Marlowe & Co, NY, 2004.

[37] Investing Answers, http://www.investinganswers.com/dictionary/income-statement

business spent (operating expenses) during this period. The P&L allows you to analyze your ability to finance expenses including repaying existing debt, financing additional debt, or reinvesting in your business, but the P&L does not show certain liabilities from non-operating costs such as business loans. Therefore, P&Ls are the basic measuring stick of (gross profit) net income after operating expenses.

Income Statement Analysis

Since the Income Statement is a report of earnings, being able to analyze income statements gives the ability to evaluate the effectiveness of the business's management of its operations.

Income Statement Importance

By thoroughly evaluating the Income Statement (P&L), you can identify where your business spends its income and compare that to similar companies in your industry. You can also compare this year's performance to the performance of past years. Remember, one important purpose of the Income Statement is to report the bottom-line profit (net income) for the year. The other main purpose is to report the total sales revenue of the business for the year and its major expenses for the year. Most importantly, however, **the Income Statement tells you whether your business is profitable or not.**

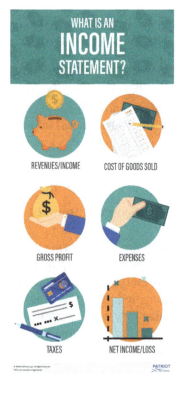

WHAT IS AN
INCOME
STATEMENT?

REVENUES/INCOME   COST OF GOODS SOLD

GROSS PROFIT   EXPENSES

TAXES   NET INCOME/LOSS

PATRIOT

88

Sample Income (P&L) Statement (annual)

All information is generated from the General Ledger.

	2017 Year to Date
Income	
4010 Private Practice Receipt	$1,896,642
4011 HealthCare Cap Payment	$470,699
4012 HealthCare Copay & Lab	$107,743
4013 BC/BS Benefits Cap Payment	$16,404
4014 Anthem Benefits Copay	$30,063
4040 Fees- Space Rental	$55,017
4220 Interest Income	$0
Total Income	**$2,576,568**
Expense	
5010 Salaries- Doctors	$479,001
5011 Salaries- Administration	$245,207
5012 Salaries- Assistants	$188,919
5013 Salaries- Other Producers	$335,021
Total Wages	**$1,248,148**
5020 Clinical Supplies	$160,538
5030 Rent & Utilities	$130,958
5040 Dues, Journals & Meetings	$3,934
5041 Advertising	$1,420
5050 Uniform Expense	$382
5060 Office Supplies	$17,652
5062 Postage	$3,830
5063 Computer MTCE & Supplies	$3,232
5064 Computer Support & Billing	$10,506
5070 Telephone	$8,115
5080 Laundry & Cleaning	$89
5090 Maintenance & Repairs	$14,676
5100 Business Insurance	$16,578
5101 Health Insurance	$44,818
5103 Life & Disability Insurance	$12,089
5110 Fees- LEGAL & Retire Plan	$4,791
5111 Fees- Accounting	$12,720
5112 Fees- Collection & Credit	$13,717
5115 Fees- Specialists	$47,008
5120 Laboratory	$147,831
5140 Interest	$9,276
5150 Payroll & Personal Prop Tax	$111,417
5160 Depreciation	$170,537
5170 401k Match- Employees	$9,698
5180 Equipment Rental	$4,268
Total Operating Expenses	**$959,854**
Total All Expenses	**$2,208,002**
7011 Officers Salaries & Benefits	$366,001
Net Inc	**$2,565**

Chart of Accounts codes are the numbers given to each type of transaction on the General Ledger.

All sources of income are listed, including interest.

Expenses are usually broken down into a Wages section and an Operating Expenses section with these two sections being added to arrive at a Total All Expenses section.

Officer's Salary and Benefits is then added near the bottom as a separate expense.

The Net Income is what is left over after adding the Total Income and subtracting the Total All Expenses and the Officers Salaries & Benefits.

©Tracker Enterprises, Inc.

Balance Sheet

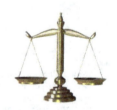

While profit-making transactions are reported in the Income Statement (P&L), a **Balance Sheet** is a financial statement that summarizes (1) a company's assets, (2) liabilities and (3) shareholders' equity at a specific point in time. These three balance sheet segments give information as to what the company owns and owes, as well as the amount invested by shareholders[38] (i.e., this is usually the healthcare professional owner). In other words, the Balance Sheet summarizes, at a particular point in time, the resources (assets) of a business on the one hand, and the obligations (liabilities) and sources of owner's equity on the other hand. The assets and liabilities reported are the results of the transactions of the business. The "transactions" are economic exchanges between the business and parties it deals with (e.g., customers, employees, vendors, etc.). As an owner and/or investor, you need to know how to examine and compare Balance Sheets in order to determine the long-term viability of your business.

The year-end and/or monthly Balance Sheet can reveal important information about the company's ability to satisfy its creditors, manage inventory, and collect its receivables.

Remember then, the Income Statement summarizes sales revenue and expenses and ends with the bottom-line profit for the period. The Balance Sheet summarizes a business's financial condition by reporting its assets, liabilities, and owners' equity at the end of the income statement period.

<u>Don't be misled by a positive P&L without understanding the Balance Sheet</u>. For example, if the practice owes money to the owner or money to a lending agency for buying or starting the practice or for getting loans for equipment purchases, these amounts do not show up in the P&L, but they do show up on the Balance Sheet.

---

[38] Investopedia. https://www.investopedia.com/terms/b/balancesheet.asp

Sample Balance Sheet (monthly)

	Oct 31, 2017
ASSETS	
Current Assets	
Checking/Savings	
1010 Cash on Hand	50.00
1030 Checking - ABC Bank	95,028.31
1031 Money Market- ABC Bank	100,266.79
Total Checking/Savings	195,345.10
Other Current Assets	
1142 Organization Cost	765.00
Total Other Current Assets	765.00
Total Current Assets	196,110.10
Fixed Assets	
1205 Current Year Fixed Assets	14,043.74
1210 Office Furniture & Equip	439,855.22
1215 Acc. Deprec Equipment	-433,037.26
1220 COMPUTER EQUIP	111,392.0
1225 Accum Depr Computer Equip.	-109,468.68
1240 Leasehold Improvements	86,170.80
1245 Amort Leasehold Improv	-29,072.00
Total Fixed Assets	79,883.82
TOTAL ASSETS	275,993.92
LIABILITIES & EQUITY	
Liabilities	
Current Liabilities	
Other Current Liabilities	
2010 Payroll Taxes- Federal	-20.89
2011 Payroll Taxes-State	2,908.68
2012 Misc. Payroll Deductions	771.31
2020 Credit Ln.	45,000.00
2020 Note- ABC Bank Credit Line	-45,000.00
2022 Note Pay- ABC Bank Computer	13,389.19
2025 Note Payable ABC Bank Tel	-586.29
2028 N/P Schein Waiting Rm Chr	-40.87
2029 Accounts Payable - Memo	32,454.49
2030 N/P CadCam	64,048.30
2033 NP ABC Bank (Laser & Cart)	19,298.46
Total Other Current Liabilities	132,222.38
Total Current Liabilities	132,222.38
Total Liabilities	132,222.38
Equity	
3040 Capital Stock	2,227.89
3041 Treasury Stock	-441,996.00
Opening Balance Equity	-3,819.93
Retained Earnings	319,634.73
Net Income	267,725.05
Total Equity	143,771.54
TOTAL LIABILITIES & EQUITY	275,993.92

All of this information is generated from the General Ledger. Definitions are from various sources and have been modified for interpretation.

Fixed Assets are long-term tangible pieces of property that a firm owns and uses in its operations to generate income. Fixed assets are not expected to be consumed or converted into cash.

Liabilities are $$ that the company owes (e.g., practice loans, mortgages, vehicle loans, equipment loans, taxes not yet paid). Don't be misled by the bottom line of the P&L since these items do NOT show up in the P&L.

Equity is that portion of the total assets that the owner or stockholders have paid for and own.

General Ledger

A **General Ledger** (GL) is a consolidated record of a company's accounting entries. The GL is the record that stores every accounting entry a company makes. The entries, called journal entries, are for both debits and credits. The entries are linked to various accounts (e.g., payroll, supplies, marketing, etc.) by account numbers (the account numbers chosen are usually done by your accountant and have no significance except as guides to each account type). These accounts fall into categories such as assets, liabilities, revenue, etc.

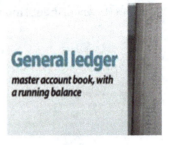

General ledger
master account book, with a running balance

A business often has dozens of accounts and thousands of journal entries in the general ledger in a year. Every journal entry should involve a debit and an offsetting credit; this is the basis of the "double-entry" bookkeeping method (i.e., the sum of all the debits in the GL should equal the sum of all the credits in the GL for a given period, which is why you might hear accountants talking about working on the "trial balance").

What else does it do? The General Ledger is what generates the income statement, balance sheet and cash flow statement.[39]

When having your accountant or bookkeeper prepare your monthly and annual General Ledger reports, ask to have the entries "detailed" or "broken down." Why? This will allow you to see how much was expensed to each vendor in specific general categories (e.g., if "Lab Expenses" is the general category, it may only show the total of all lab expenses, but the detailed version would be a breakdown of all the different vendors under the Lab Expenses. Also, request "splits" for your credit card expenses since this will show the breakdown on what is expensed for each credit card and for whom.

---

[39] Investing Answers. http://www.investinganswers.com/financial-dictionary/businesses-corporations/general-ledger-5978

Small Sampling a General Ledger (monthly)

> The General Ledger is where all chart of accounts originate.

Date	Ref	Description	Balance	Debit	Credit	Total
	5061 Technology Support		3,229.89			
08/10/15	21343	Patterson Dental Supply, Inc.		315.74		
08/13/15	21360	U.S. BANK-timeclick support call		59.00		
08/06/15	JE.006	Cardmember Service-dexis 6/19 support		451.71		
08/06/15	JE.006	Cardmember Service-henry schein hardware support		104.55		
08/06/15	JE.006	Cardmember Service-dexis 7/20 support		451.71		
				1,382.71	0.00	4,612.60
	5063 Postage		2,575.01			
08/05/15	21338	PURCHASE POWER		402.50		
				402.50	0.00	2,977.51
	5070 Telephone		3,304.16			
08/13/15	21357	TDS METROCOM		439.20		
				439.20	0.00	3,743.36
	5071 Cellular Phone		338.63			
				0.00	0.00	338.63
	5074 Website Fees		2,452.50			
				0.00	0.00	2,452.50
	5080 Laundry & Cleaning		548.07			
				0.00	0.00	548.07
	5090 Office Equip Repair & Maint		16.00			
08/13/15	21360	U.S. BANK·				
				1,575.00		
				1,575.00	0.00	1,591.00

> This is a fictitious copy of only a small part of a many-paged detailed General Ledger.

Statement of Cash Flows

The **Statement of Cash Flows** reports how much cash was generated from profit and the other sources of cash, and what the business did with this money. In other words, it demonstrates the cash that moves through your business in the form of receipts, expenses, and capital expenditures. It represents the cash required to keep your business operating on a day-to-day basis. Projecting cash flow tells you how much money you need to run the business, i.e., how much is needed to pay the bills. It *focuses* on the sources and uses of cash during a given time period and *asks* where the business got its money and what it did with it? Since the business often needs other sources of cash besides profit, the Statement of Cash Flows discloses whether the business raised additional capital during the year, whether it made major capital expenditures (investments in fixed assets) during the year, and whether it distributed money from profit to its owners. If nothing else, it reveals what a business did with the cash from its profit. [40]

A Statement of Cash Flows measures the sources of a company's cash (whereas the Income Statement measures a company's financial performance). It shows exactly how much money a company has received and how much it has spent, traditionally over a period of one month. It captures the current operating results and changes on the balance sheet such as increases or decreases in accounts receivable or accounts payable and does not include noncash accounting such as depreciation and amortization. A cash flow statement is used to determine the short-term viability and liquidity of a company, specifically how well it is positioned to pay its bills and vendors.[41]

---

[40] Tracy, John A., Accounting for Dummies (3rd Ed), Wiley Publishing Inc, 2005.

[41] Investopedia, https://www.investopedia.com/ask/answers/031215/what-difference-between-cash-flow-statement-and-income-statement.asp

Income Statements differ from Cash Flow Statements

An income statement (P&L) shows how much money your business makes and spends within a given time period. It summarizes how your business earned revenue, paid expenses, and arrived at its bottom line.

A cash flow statement shows the incomings and outgoings of your business's cash within a given time period. This type of report typically divides cash by use.

- **Financing:** Cash used for borrowing and lending
- **Operations:** Cash used during daily operations
- **Investing:** Cash used to purchase equipment or other assets

Should you view the P&L or the Cash Flow Statement?

When we work with our healthcare professional clients, we believe that the Income Statement (P&L), Balance Sheet and General Ledger provide the bigger picture. They account for financial factors beyond cash flow, including non-cash expenses such as depreciation, and allow you to observe your business's longer-term trends in spending and earning.

Your income statement can help you better answer questions such as: How did my business perform last year? Where can I cut back on costs?[42]

---

[42] Wells Fargo Works for Small Business.
https://wellsfargoworks.com/management/article/understanding-income-statements-and-cash-flow-statements

If you don't have the info, you can't make the decisions

Knowledge is Power.
Sir Francis Bacon

I see the following circumstances occur too frequently. Typically, financial statements are prepared, at best, on a quarterly basis, and in some instances, only once per year. This can be a disaster waiting to happen. Imagine this sample scenario assuming your statements are only done once per quarter. Let's assume we are discussing the first quarter (e.g., January 1 - March 31):

- Bank statements come in (statements can be accessed as early as the day after the end of the month from the Internet).
- It takes 2 weeks to assemble information (now it's April 15th).
- 10 days later, the accountant receives the info (by April 25th).
- If you're lucky, the accountant gets to them immediately, but what if it's quarterly tax time or annual tax season? If that's the case, the accountant may not get to them until after tax season.
- The accountant starts working on your financials May 1; it takes a week to complete the financials.
- You receive the completed financials a week later (May 15th).
- You look at them 2 weeks later (June 1st), if you look at all.

> *Because it has taken you too long to react*, you may now be on a trend from which you may not be able to recover.

It's now 5 months after the year started; you finally received statistics on your first quarter finances. What if, in January, a trend started where you *spent too much* and *made too little*?

> *You need to know more about your finances, and you need to know in a more timely fashion.*

To avoid this scenario, you must be able to compare, *in a timely fashion and on a regular basis*, the current month, quarter, and annual financials, and, most importantly, update your actual and predicted revenue and expenses. Then, you can make adjustments, as needed, to stay on a successful path to your goals.

You need a system ...

You now understand the *cost in time* involved in preparing all of the information you need to analyze your financial status.[43] In addition, owners have to develop some knowledge on how to read their financial statements.

> *To be successful*, you need to be able to see the results of your decisions before you act on them.

You will also need a system that periodically updates you on your practice's progress and allows you to make financial decisions with confidence. It is recommended you have your financials prepared on a monthly basis whether by your accountant, bookkeeper, office manager, etc. Then, <u>meet with your accountant quarterly to review and update your tax situation</u>. You need to know that your choices are based on solid facts so that you can then concentrate on what you really started out to do, being a healthcare provider.

Start thinking about what the following chart might suggest. Then, read **Section IV: Optimizing**.

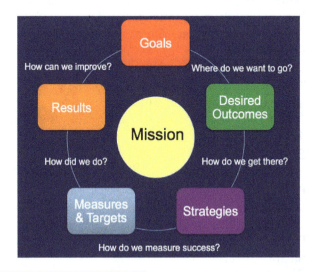

---

[43] Small Business Sourcebook. Gale Publishing. ISBN-13: 9780787657628

Expand Summary

1. Why you need to understand basic business principles to excel in your practice.
2. Where are you, Where are you going, Where have you been?
3. What is the Optimal Business Management system?
   a. Planning
   b. Monitoring
   c. Analyzing
   d. Anticipating
   e. Improving
4. Consider monitoring these statistics:
   a. Production
   b. Revenue
   c. Accounts receivables
   d. Provider statistics
   e. Labor costs including salaries and benefits
   f. All expenses including debt service
   g. Scheduling
   h. Patient information statistics
5. The three job descriptions you have
   a. Entrepreneur
   b. Manager (Owner)
   c. Technician
6. Understanding business terminology
   a. Production
   b. Revenue
   c. Expenses
   d. Net Income
   e. Profit
   f. Cash Flow
7. Understanding financial reports
   a. Profit and Loss Statements (P&L)/Income Statements
   b. Balance Sheets
   c. General Ledgers
   d. Cash Flow Statements

Expand Action Plan: The Road Map

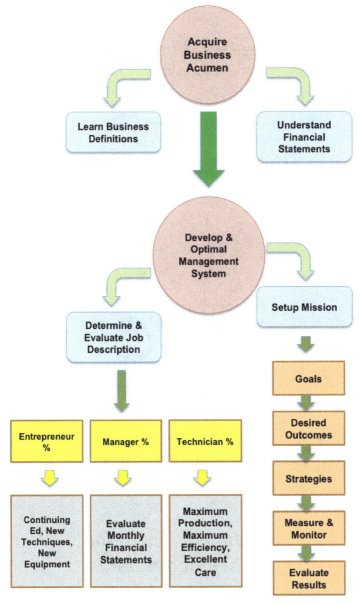

©Tracker Enterprises, Inc.

Question Everything!
Albert Einstein

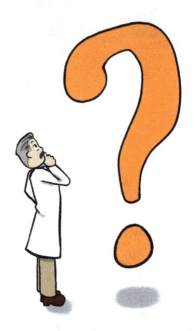

*Knowledge is having
the right answer.*

*Intelligence is asking
the right question.*

SECTION IV: OPTIMIZE

CHAPTER 16: MY STORY CONTINUES TO IMPROVE

I was seeing a lot of patients and realizing some big checks every month from HMOs and PPOs. I had two doctors working for me and seventeen staff – all necessary for the workload. Money was good, but hours and pace were brutal (for everyone). It was time to start optimizing my practice – making it the best it could be.

I started by seriously considering my concerns about working with many of my HMO and PPO patients because they just didn't seem to have the motivation for getting the best treatment; they just wanted the cheapest treatment. They also rarely said, *"Thanks, Doc, you did a great job"* or, *"I'm so happy with what you did for me."* My patients who paid the usual and customary fees for treatment, however, were thankful and appreciative – go figure! To give you an example, one group of patients we treated only had to pay $2.00 (that's two dollars) per appointment because they were covered by a state-sanctioned, union-supported HMO. Some of these patients actually complained that they should not have had to pay the $2.00 fee.

You get what you pay for.

Unfortunately, spending quality time with patients had become more difficult because I was unable to control the big staff and patient load. In addition, without my knowledge, cheaper supplies were being ordered to keep down costs since we didn't make as much per procedure as we had in the past.

No matter how many doctors I had helping me or how many staff we had to support us, everyone in the office was on roller skates five to six days per week with typical overtime occurring for most of the staff. The time I should have been spending as a Manager and Entrepreneur had been completely overshadowed by my need to be a Technician.

The last straw occurred when my office manager said: *"We need to have a meeting, doc."* She told me that full-paying patients who wanted to schedule an appointment for high-dollar procedures were being told that the first available appointment was in three months. I did some calculations - even without the large capitation and PPO checks received every month, I could make more money by no longer accepting HMO and PPO patients and by opening my schedule to regular, fee-for-service patients. Plus, I could cut my staff including one doctor. I went cold turkey and resigned from all of those programs. I was scared to death that the loss of the monthly cap checks would kill my revenue stream. I was back staring at the ceiling again.

My fears were alleviated when the revenue without those HMO and PPO patients was $10,000 more than before. On top of that, I was saving $5,000 to $10,000 per month in labor costs and clinical supplies. That settled it; I never looked back.

My situation doesn't apply to every practice. I have consulted with some large practices that accept HMO and PPO with checks averaging $50,000 or more per month. The staff size and overhead appeared overwhelming, but the owner was taking home huge salaries – much larger than the average practitioner. Some of these owners managed to still see patients, but their patient load was usually very minimal. Instead, they placed emphasis on the Manager slice of the pie discussed in the previous chapter. I continue to caution them that insurance programs have a tendency to change over the years. For example, a large CAP program, when they do their annual planning, might decide to switch their provider-base to other providers. If this happens, the owner might experience a significant cash flow problem without the ability to make payroll for the larger staff, pay rent for the larger space, or pay for the excess equipment he already has to provide for a large patient base.

Once I was back to what I considered a normal practice for me -- seeing the patients I wanted to see and those that wanted the right treatment for their conditions (and who were willing to pay for it), I decided I was on the right track. I wanted to continue improving (optimizing) my practice.

Since I now had a good feel for understanding my monthly financial statements, I decided to take the next step in taking control of the finances. I wanted to prepare for the future. I spent a considerable amount of time discussing my goals with a good friend (he had the qualifications since he was a former chief financial executive for one of the world's largest computer manufacturers). In order to assist me, he offered to help me prepare a budget for the next year. Together, we developed a spreadsheet and analysis software program that allowed me to enter all of the previous year's production, revenue, expenses and liabilities. He then recommended we take this one step further. We then developed a "forecasting" program that allowed me to take information from the static budget and convert it to the actual ongoing new financial information that came in each month. This also allowed me to do what if scenarios and reformat the year going forward after each month's actual information was received. I could accurately predict how the practice would do as the year progressed and then make the necessary adjustments in production and expenses to meet or exceed my annual goals.

All of a sudden, I was able to adjust my production rate, order new equipment, hire new staff, increase staff benefits, take the expensive continuing education courses I desired, and adjust my own salary and benefits with the confidence that I was making my decisions based on sound financial statistics that were available to me. I paid my initial loans off. Unexpected expenses, however, always occur. Existing equipment became obsolete; new equipment was purchased with new loans; more loans were paid off; continuing education prompted new equipment that required new loans. But, with my new knowledge and ability to readjust my revenue and expenses, the loans were easily paid off. Success was great, but it resulted in the need for a larger space and satellite offices and more equipment; new loans were required. I designed and built a beautiful new office with the best equipment and the best staff. I built a satellite office. More loans were paid off. I had control.

Life was good.

*When Alice reached a fork in the road,
she asked the Cheshire cat which way she should go.
He asked her where she was going.
Alice replied that she didn't know.
The cat concluded matter-of-factly,
"Then it doesn't matter which way you go."*[44]

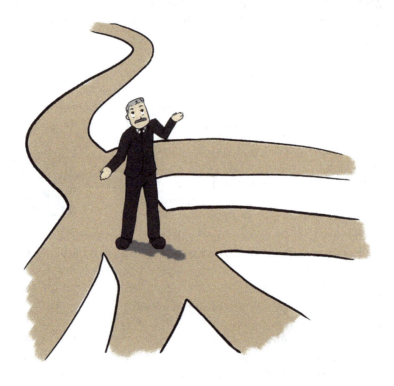

---

[44] Carroll, Lewis. Alice in Wonderland, ISBN-13: 978-0393932348

Chapter 17: Your Story - Take the Right Path

Are you ready to be more successful?

If all you are provided with are stale, historical financial reports without receiving a clear opinion on the future financial status of your business, you need to supplement your financial reports with a financial forecasting tool that does. If your existing information doesn't offer the ability to do "what if" scenarios, you need a tool that does. If you are used to being provided with accounting reports but not evaluations of those reports, you need a tool that gives you information in a language you understand and in a format so that you can evaluate the financial status of your practice in less than one hour per month. These components are part of an ideal Optimal Operational Management tool that will allow you to see if you are *progressing* as planned.

You need to be open to going through a transformation, because transformation shifts you from a less resourceful and valuable state to a more resourceful and valuable state. Take a leap of faith; make a transformation. Begin the process of understanding your financial reports and monitoring your practice management software statistics. Then you will have the information you need to adjust for the future.

My upcoming recommendations to consider understanding more about your business operations include suggestions meant to improve your chances for immediate and long-term success. By using these optimized business principles, your chances for success, or greater success than you already have, can improve dramatically. This is a template for success that can *significantly increase* the chances that your business investment will continue to appreciate.

> **Use proper tools for the job.**

*Information is the
Gatekeeper to Success*

*Those who are unaware
that they are walking in darkness
will never seek the light.*[45]

Or, more bluntly,

*What you don't know
can and will hurt you.*

---

[45] Lee, Bruce

What is the optimal model to manage your practice?

My goal is to stimulate you to think how successful CEOs run their businesses. Simply put, their success stories revolve around how they understand their businesses (i.e., how their businesses operate). I urge you to take a leap of faith; take on a larger role as a Manager. Learn how you can better understand what the information you have available through your financial reports and the office statistics provided by your practice management software are trying to tell you. When you understand this information, you will be able to dynamically adjust your practice for every opportunity and obstacle that arises.

By standard definition, **Optimal Operational Management** refers to the administration of business practices to create the highest level of efficiency possible within an organization. It includes the design and control of operations that convert resources into desired goods and services and implements a business strategy to maximize profit. It involves the delivery of goods and services to customers within the agreed time commitment, and then follows up with customers to ensure the products/services meet customers' quality and functionality needs. Finally, Optimal Operational Management takes the feedback received and distributes the relevant information to the business owner and team to use in improvement.[46]

For your purposes, **Optimal Operational Management** is the process of taking actual, real-time financial numbers and re-forecasting them into a format that is made up of all the different parameters and components of production, revenue and expenses in order to demonstrate past,

> Optimal Operational Management is the monitoring, measuring, analyzing, and adjusting of the operations of a practice in order to best manage the expectations of the patients and goals of the doctor/owner.

[46] Investopedia, https://www.investopedia.com/terms/o/operations-management.asp

present and future income and expenses. Once you have actual financial information (i.e., financial reports from your accountant) for a given time period that has already happened, you should be able to better predict where you are headed; the remainder of the year needs to be filled in with forecasted (predicted) numbers. Analysis (monitoring, measuring, redirecting and implementing) should constantly be done on this combination of actuals and forecasts to see how well the practice is doing, at any point in time, and how well the practice will do as the year progresses. After analyzing where your practice is at present and what it did in the past, you can alter the forecasts to redirect you to the path you need to take to reach your goals.

The Ingredients to Optimal Operational Management

- Ensuring that business operations are designed in terms of meeting customer (i.e., patient) requirements.
- Acquiring the skills and understanding of the financial and other operational information required for success.
- Managing the process that converts inputs into outputs.
  - Inputs are the production, revenue, expenses, customers, staff, and statistics or key performance indicators (KPIs).
  - Outputs are the products, services, customers, and goals.
  - Making improvements along the way.

The following illustration represents how Optimal Operational Management cycles work according to the above principles:

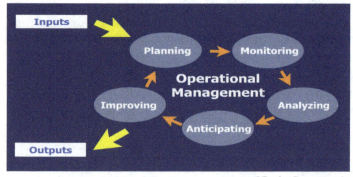

©Tracker Enterprises, Inc. 2018

You need to breakdown monitoring further by looking at resources from the areas indicated in the following two charts. The following statistics are usually readily available from your practice management software. Since monitoring these statistics is key to your understanding of how your business is doing, they are often referred to as Key Performance Indicators (KPIs).

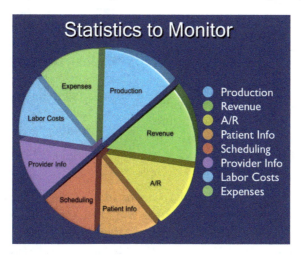

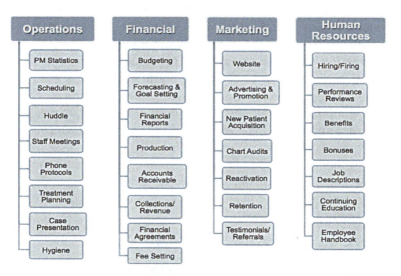

What do you need to make smart financial decisions?

To optimize your practice's financial outlook, you need a model that is easy to use so that you can analyze what happens to production, revenue, expenses, and profits when key factors that drive your business are exposed to changes, anticipated or not. Remember, you need to be able to plan for how you will close the gap between historical revenue and expense information received from your accountant and proposed future information you obtain through Optimal Operational Management.

> While accounting provides the financial information and analysis tools you need for analyzing past performance, *forecasting gives you the ability to 'try out' anticipated decisions.*

Since your accountant is set up to analyze past numbers and is not set up to forecast the future, you need a tool that allows you to quickly see the problem areas and then provide the information needed to make predictable decisions based on sound forecasting. Accounting reports (P&Ls, Balance Sheets, General Ledgers, Statements of Cash Flow, etc.) are essential to analyze where you've been, but they provide only historical information. You need a model that provides for ongoing actual statistics and then allows for future predictions. Also, a good useable model should be easily viewed, should provide all pertinent information (historical and predicted) in a way that is both *easily* understood (even if you don't have an accounting background), and also viewable *without taking up too much of your valuable time*. With the correct model, you should be able to evaluate the health of your practice in one hour or less each month and then, make the recommendations to readjust the forecasting going forward.

Take to heart this quote from Thomas Jefferson:

> ***I like the dreams of the future***
> ***better than the history of the past.***

Built in controls ...

Only bad things happen quickly.[47]

Don't be caught with unexpected expenses that can't be offset by revenue. Alarm capabilities must be built into your model. For example, actual revenue and expenses must be compared with predicted revenue and expenses. Serious variances need to set off red flags so that you can deal with them before they become major problems.

> Your financial planning tools need to show you *where you've been, where you are, and most importantly, where you're going.*

The history of things to come ...

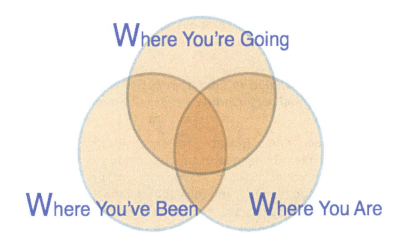

©Tracker Enterprises, Inc. 2018

Every "Where" has to mesh with every other "Where."

---

[47]Livingston, Gordon. *Too Soon Old, Too Late Smart,* Marlowe & Co, NY, 2004.

Are you asking the right questions?

Your model needs to have a checklist of key questions to ask. Imagine that if you are planning to invest in a another business or have already invested money in the business, their financial tools should provide answers as to how the company is doing, how it will most likely do in the future, and whether you should consider putting your hard-earned cash into their company.

Therefore, you need to ask the right questions. Your financial forecasting tool should help you answer the following questions:

- Is the practice experiencing unusual gains or losses?
- Are profits holding or improving?
- Are profits keeping pace with expenses?
- How does income compare to expenses?
- Are changes in assets and liabilities consistent with the growth needed?
- Are there any signs of financial distress?
- Are there any unusual liabilities?

> *Making a profit* should be the main financial goal of your business.

Knowledge without application is useless.
All good performance starts with clear goals.
Ken Blanchard

This ideal Optimal Business Management model needs to be able to take the existing historical information available from financial reports provided by your accountant, present it to you in a way you understand, and then allow you to predict (or forecast) where the practice will be in the future. If the predictions are not ideal, you should be able to make changes with a forecasting tool that allows you to predict a better outcome and what you will need to do to get there.

The next few chapters are designed to help you better understand what Budgets and Forecasts can provide to you to allow for a more successful business outcome going forward.

What would this Optimal Management tool look like?

The ideal Optimal Business Management tool would contain:

1. A tool that allows you to prepare an annual Budget.
2. A tool that allows you to do What If scenarios.
3. A tool that allows you to reforecast the months going forward after receiving the information in monthly reports provided by the accountant and practice software.
4. A tool that shows Key Performance Indicator statistics (KPIs) for monitoring and measuring progress.
5. A tool that provides spreadsheets and written analyses each month to allow you to view your practice's financial status in one hour or less per month.

An in depth explanation of how to prepare an Optimal Business Management model is beyond the scope of this book. If you would like us to help you assemble this highly advantageous tool, ask me about what we offer and how we can help you by emailing me at pjp@trackerenterprises.com. If, on the other hand, you do not have the time or interest to prepare your own Optimal Business Management model, or you are not interested in entering the information in the model and arriving at an Analysis, we can prepare that model for you and then enter the information and analyze it for you on a monthly basis. Let us know what works best for you.

We didn't actually overspend our budget. The allocations simply fell short of our expenditures.
Keith Davis

Chapter 18: Who Needs A Budget, Anyway?

"My problem is reconciling my gross habits
with my net income."
Errol Flynn

Most of us doctors can relate to the witty quote above by the playboy movie star, Errol Flynn (1909 – 1959). Not that we have any "gross habits," but we tend to sometimes allow our whims, not hard evidence, to dictate our spending habits.

> The old days are gone when a doctor could "hang a shingle" and be successful in spite of the doctor's efforts, or lack thereof.

Owners who are exceptionally good in business aren't necessarily good because of what they know but because of their voracious need to know more. The problem with most failing businesses is not that the owners do not know enough about clinical care or marketing, but that they spend very little time and energy understanding their financials. [48]

At one of my recent seminars, I asked the 40 participants for a show of hands for those that did annual budgets; only one doctor responded that he did. Only 8 doctors said that they understood what a budget was. Do you do a budget? Successful companies do budgets once per year. If you have not yet done a budget, it is time to consider it.

> The *best* business owners *learn what it takes* to succeed.

Take the first steps to knowing exactly
where your practice is going financially.
Prepare a budget.

---

[48] Gerber, Michael E. The E-Myth, p. xv. HarperCollins Publishers, Inc., 1995.

What is a Budget?

A **Budget** is a plan that outlines an organization's financial and operational goals. It may be thought of as an action plan for the future. Planning a budget helps a business allocate resources, evaluate performance, and formulate plans. Its main use is to predict your practice's ability to take in more cash than it pays out.[49] Budgeting (often incorrectly referred to as being one and the same as forecasting) is the periodic (typically annual) review of past (historic) financial information with the sole purpose of estimating future financial conditions and creating a fiscal plan of revenues and expenses that can then be managed to for that specific period of time.[50]

> It would be difficult to apply past knowledge for practical use if there wasn't a history, or road map, of the knowledge in the first place.

The budget is also an essential part of a business plan when starting a new business. Once a business is established, budgeting should become a regular task that occurs on an annual basis, where the past year's budget and actual performance are reviewed and analyzed and then, new budget projections are made for the next year.

Budgets are good for planning for the future by looking at the past. For example, what did you do last year and how might those financial experiences apply to the next year, and what new expenses or new sources of revenue may occur?

---

[49] Ward, Susan. The Balance. https://www.thebalance.com/business-budget-2948312

[50] Tyson, Eric. Small Business for Dummies (2nd Ed). Wiley Publishing Inc, 2003.

Why should you consider a budget for your practice?

In order for your business to achieve maximum success, dependable budgets are necessary for sound planning. Budgets help to define and predict production and revenue information and dollar requirements for areas such as labor (hiring, raises, etc.), clerical and clinical supplies, laboratory costs, rent or mortgage expenses, capital expenses (equipment and maintenance, etc.), communications, administration, marketing, the development of new products and services and/or changes proposed for existing products or services, leasehold improvements and servicing debt.

A comprehensive budget will also be a definite requirement for obtaining business loans from financial institutions. If you are planning on starting a practice, preparing a budget plays an important role in determining your start up and operating costs.

Making budget estimates ...

It is important to be realistic with your budget projections, particularly if you are starting a new business and have no previous year's budget figures to guide your estimates. There are often radical differences between actual and projected revenues and expenses due to unforeseen changes such as:

- Gaining/losing patients resulting in changing revenue
- Having to purchase or replace equipment
- Increases in rent and other fixed expenses
- Hiring employees or increasing salaries and/or benefits

Your financial reports (e.g., Income or P&L Statements, Balance Sheets, General Ledgers, etc.) are designed to demonstrate how your business has performed in the past so that you can use this information to guide you in assembling your budget for the next year.

Once you have evaluated last year's performance from historically based financial reports, you can redirect that information toward the preparation of your budget.

Reasons for budgeting ...

Budgets should be done for 3 reasons: modeling, planning, and control.

1. *Modeling*

You will need the following information to prepare your budget blueprint or model:

> The Budget should be a model, or blueprint, that serves as the foundation of your business future.

- Last year's Income statements
- Balance sheets from last year
- General ledgers from last year

2. *Planning*

One of the main purposes of budgeting is to develop a definite and detailed achievable financial plan for the upcoming period. To construct a budget, you have to establish explicit financial objectives for the coming year and then identify exactly what has to be done to accomplish these financial goals. It should answer the following questions:

- How are you going to get there from here?
- Will it allow you to pass that vision, on paper, to your team?
- Does the Budget impose deadlines for achieving the goals?

3. *Control*

The budget plan is used like a map to keep you on course. Significant variations, as the year progresses, raise red flags so that you can make the necessary corrections to get you back on course. Remember not to change numbers in the budget; change numbers in the forecast (more on this in the next chapter). The budget should be used only as a guide for the upcoming year and for a grading tool to help you do better in your budget planning for the next year.

A budget has these additional advantages:

- It forces you to do better estimating by compelling you to reevaluate past performance to identify changes.
- It provides tools for evaluating your and your team's performance, and it incentivizes everyone to shoot for goals.

There are two ways to budget from year to year:

1. **Assume a percentage increase** (e.g., 5%) for each fixed expense category (e.g., rent), each variable expense category (e.g., supplies), and each revenue category. *I am not a fan of this method since it bases expense and revenue increases on percentages that have no actual basis in reality. I feel more comfortable with a system based on actual historical data.*
2. **Zero-based budgeting** assumes that the budgeting process starts with new values each year. For example, you budget based on past experience and estimated future needs. *This is the method I prefer.*

No matter which system you use, the important thing is that you choose one and then plan for the future year as accurately as possible. This gives you a base, or starting point, to help you determine how much revenue will be needed to meet expenses and provide for profit.

Remember that budgets are a view of past reality based on historical information that may be valid for only a very short period of time – usually quickly fading in accuracy as new realities evolve. Budgeting is not a crystal ball or wishful thinking; it must start with a broad-based analysis of the most recent historical performance and position of the business. Then, you must decide on specific and reachable goals for the upcoming year.

> *Do not* think of a Budget as more than it really is.

You can do budgets for as many years (e.g., 1, 2, 3, 5, etc.) into the future as you want, but your most accurate budget will come if you do it one year at a time. Estimating for twelve months is hard enough, so it's usually best to stick with a one-year budget.

The exception is when you need to provide a 3 - 5 year Budget for a Business Plan presentation to a lending institution or investors.

Why some practices avoid budgeting ...

It is common for healthcare professionals to not do budgeting at all. Reasons include:

If you believe chaos is in control, attempting to predict the future may seem futile.

- Many doctors are comfortable with past profits and status quo, so they see no value in spending the time or costs involved in preparing budgets.
- Owners accept fate and hope for the best, usually because the practice has been somewhat successful in the past in spite of its lack of financial organization.
- Owners lack the expertise necessary to prepare a budget.
- Someone in the practice (e.g., an office manager) takes on the responsibility of establishing internal accounting reports and tells the owner/doctor that budgets will not be necessary.

The importance of detailed budgets ...

Business owners need to carefully analyze how their actions (price setting for services, purchasing supplies and equipment, hiring employees, etc.) might impact profit before making final decisions. Understand that each decision carries numerous ancillary consequences with it. For example, hiring a new employee does not simply include that employee's salary, but it may also include the following financial consequences:

- Payroll and unemployment taxes
- Retirement benefits
- Uniform allowances
- Holiday and sick pay
- Bonuses
- Health insurance
- SUTA and FUTA
- Gifts, continuing education, travel, lodging expenses, etc.

Information you will need to prepare a budget …

1. ***Production information***. Remember, production is what
   your practice charges out for procedures you and your other
   producers/providers (e.g., associate doctors, PAs, physical
   therapists, hygienists, etc.) do. You should start by estimating
   what each provider's charges might be in the new year. A
   good way to do this is to take the average daily production
   per provider for the most recently completed year. Once you
   know that, and you know the number of days each provider
   will work in the coming year; simply do the math. Example:

Name	Title	Days Worked Last Yr	Total Production Last Year	Production per Day Last Year	Days Proposed This Year	Anticipated Production per Day	Anticipated Annual Production
Dr. Smith	Associate Dr	160	$400,000	$2,500	168	$2,500	$420,000

©Tracker Enterprises, Inc. 2018

2. ***Revenue information*** consists of the <u>actual dollars collected</u>
   for the production your practice earns. <u>Remember, revenue,
   not production, pays the bills</u>. Ideally, revenue should relate
   directly to your production estimates, but in most practices,
   these values will not be the same. The following are examples
   of why these values may differ:

   - Are your accounts receivable programs in order? If you
     have high accounts receivables, especially in the over 90-
     day category, revenue will never compare well with
     production.

   - Your practice accepts alternative insurance (e.g., PPOs,
     HMOs, etc.)? If so, you will have to adjust the revenue
     anticipated based on the percentage discounts you might
     expect from these alternative insurance plans. For
     example, if the total production this year was $1,400,000
     and the total revenue was $980,000, you can assume your
     revenue for the next year will be approximately 70% of
     the proposed production. Unless you exit some
     alternative insurance plans, this will not improve.

Example:

Total Production Last Year	Total Revenue Last Year	% of Revenue to Production	Anticipated Annual Revenue Needed This Year	Anticipated Production Needed To Meet Revenue
$1,400,000	$980,000	70%	$1,100,000	$1,571,400

©Tracker Enterprises, Inc. 2018

3. ***Expenses information*** includes the everyday costs of running your practice, your personal compensation, liability expenses, debt service, etc. As indicated before, there are two basic approaches to budget your expenses from year to year:

- The first way is to *assume a percentage increase* for each expense. By adding a percentage to last year's values, you can arrive at next year's budget rapidly. *Remember, this method gives a quick but not very accurate estimate.*

Example:

Expense Name	Total Expense Last Year	% Increase Expected	Anticipated Expense This Year
Staff Salaries & Benefits	$320,000	5.00%	$336,000
Clinical Supplies	$66,000	4.00%	$68,640
Clerical Supplies	$44,000	4.00%	$45,760

©Tracker Enterprises, Inc. 2018

- If you want to estimate your expenses more accurately, you might want to consider a more in-depth evaluation. *Zero-based budgeting* assumes that each new budget year's expenses start at zero. For example, with clinical supplies, you would assume, based on past experience and estimated future needs, how much will be used in the next year; you could get bids from different suppliers to determine if you've been getting the best deals in the past or if their prices will be increasing by a certain percentage in the new year.

One word of advice: the idea of ordering supplies at a discount because you order in advance for 3, 6 or 12 months is no longer the norm. Order what you need when you need it. <u>Run lean and mean</u>. You will save in the long run since you will save on losses incurred in not using supplies before the expiration dates or simply ordering more than you needed.

Example:

Expense Name	Total Expense Last Year	Actual Increase Expected	Anticipated Expense This Year
Staff Salaries & Benefits	$320,000	$34,000	$354,000
Clinical Supplies	$66,000	$7,500	$73,500
Clerical Supplies	$44,000	$4,100	$48,100

©Tracker Enterprises, Inc. 2018

Once you have determined your production, revenue and expenses, it becomes a simple matter of mathematics. Subtract the anticipated expenses from the revenue to determine your profitability. If the outcome is negative, you need to make adjustments to increase production and revenue to offset expenses, or you need to decrease expenses, or a combination of both.

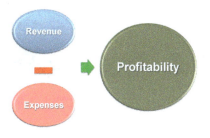

Example:

Total Revenue Expected	Total Expenses Expected	Profit Expected
$1,100,000	$840,000	$260,000

©Tracker Enterprises, Inc. 2018

What adjustments might you consider if expected revenue is less than the expenses or less than what you desire for profit:

- Add days to provider/producer schedules to add production
- Increase fees
- Decrease holes in the schedules
- Decrease expenses
- Collect on accounts receivable in a more timely fashion and recover overdue accounts receivable
- Etc., etc.

Remember, once the Budget is completed, it is not meant to be dynamic. It is only used as a visualization of what is predicted for the year. Actual expenses and revenue will constantly evolve.

Hierarchy of budgeting ...

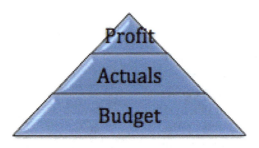

©Tracker Enterprises, Inc. 2018

Traditionally, budgets have been visualized as seen in the triangle above. The base of the triangle is the **Budget** since it is the foundation from which all other actions are built. The middle section shows the **Actuals**; these are the expenses and revenue that have actually happened as the year progresses and obviously will be different from those originally estimated in the budget. The problem is in the section labeled **Profit**. Initially, this might look okay, but what if the following occurs: the **Actuals** show you under-estimated your expenses or overestimated your revenue – i.e., you are spending too much or taking in too little.

If you agree that the dynamically changing **Actuals** and **Profit** are not really connected to the static **Budget**, then a better representation is shown in the following figure.

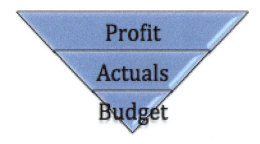

©Tracker Enterprises, Inc. 2018

Remember, your **Budget** was done from figures from last year and was, therefore, based on what had already occurred. In reality, any unforeseen economic event can cause the triangle to lean one direction or another, or worse, collapse. If it starts to lean, the top section (**Profit**) needs to slide in the opposite direction to maintain some form of balance. The more it leans, the more the change in the **Profit** needs to be, all because of what was your best guess (your **Budget**) at one point in time. Then, the following questions become inevitable:

- *Can* I make good decisions when the Budget is leaning?
- *Can* the leaning be stopped?
- *Why* didn't I get some advanced notice?
- *Why* don't I know what to expect next?
- *Why* didn't my expert advisors let me know?
- *How* will I cope with these surprises?

Unfortunately, in addition to using a Budget as a starting point for estimating what might happen, most owners make the mistake of trying to use it throughout the year. Since unpredicted financial events occur constantly, relying only on a budget alone almost guarantees that the best decision at any point in time is almost impossible to make. In other words, how can you estimate the changes you need to make as the year progresses if the Budget is static and does not show what is actually happening?

Remember, a Budget is only a "stake in the ground," and it's history. History tells what has already happened and makes us consider what we might expect, but it <u>doesn't show what will actually occur in the future, and it does not allow for adjustments</u>.

Sample Healthcare Professional Budget ...

The following chart is an example of what a summary of a Budget might look like for a healthcare professional. Understand that values shown are summaries of categories that have come from detailed breakdowns of General Ledger and P&L information from the previous year. This is a summary page. In reality, you would arrive at this summary from a detailed budget preparation. It is not important whether your Budget looks like this example; it is important that it contains input from every possible source of Production, Revenue and Expenses. This particular sample does not contain other information that will be on the Balance Sheet.

BUDGET SUMMARY REPORT

DR. JOHN SAMPLE

BUDGET Summary	JAN BUD	FEB BUD	MAR BUD	APRIL BUD	MAY BUD	JUNE BUD	JULY BUD	AUG BUD	SEPT BUD	OCT BUD	NOV BUD	DEC BUD	YEAR BUD
PRODUCTION													
DOCTOR OWNER	100000	90000	100000	96000	100000	92000	96000	96000	92000	100000	90000	90000	1142000
DOCTOR ASSOCIATE	66800	61350	62150	65300	69050	59100	58250	63400	54900	70800	62500	57950	751550
PRODUCTS FOR RESALE	2213	2213	2213	2213	2213	2213	2213	2213	2213	2213	2213	2213	26556
TOTAL PRODUCTION	169013	153563	164363	163513	171263	153313	156463	161613	149113	173013	154713	150163	1920106
REVENUE													
SERVICES	143661	130529	139709	138986	145574	130316	132994	137371	126746	147061	131506	127639	1632090
MISC. INCOME OTHER	450	450	450	450	450	450	450	450	450	450	450	450	5400
ADJUSTMENTS TO INCOME	(836)	(836)	(836)	(836)	(836)	(836)	(836)	(836)	(836)	(836)	(836)	(836)	(10032)
TOTAL REVENUE	143275	130143	139323	138600	145188	129930	132608	136985	126360	146675	131120	127253	1627458
EXPENSES													
STAFF PAY & BENEFITS	49426	46112	56460	48631	47957	46173	44534	56146	43024	49158	45183	44172	576977
ASSOCIATE COMP	16700	15338	15538	16325	17263	14775	14563	15850	13725	17700	15625	14488	187888
CAPITAL & FACILITIES	6054	6750	8237	5754	6213	6204	6476	6204	8187	6104	4978	5254	76415
LAB	12000	12000	12000	12000	12000	12000	12000	12000	12000	12000	12000	12000	144000
SUPPLIES	16086	14321	14571	15931	14571	14316	16081	14316	14666	15831	14566	14316	179572
ADMINISTRATIVE	8700	5463	6823	6825	5463	6057	10266	5463	6923	9700	7463	6057	85202
MARKETING	6000	6000	6000	6000	6000	6000	6000	6000	6000	6000	6000	6000	72000
SUBTOTAL EXPENSES	114966	105983	119628	111466	109466	105525	109919	115979	104525	116493	105815	102287	1322053
TOTAL OP EXPENSES	96697	90146	103060	93572	91704	90169	93788	99629	89769	98836	88621	86768	1122759
TOTAL OP PROFIT	35751	2356	28150	40757	45447	34656	26830	35294	30898	46778	42935	33652	403404

Sample preparation included the following information:

- The Owner and Associate Doctor production estimates came from the previous year's average production per day times the number of days estimated to be worked in the next year.
- Revenue was estimated to be 85% of production based on collected revenue/production averages for the previous year.
- Expenses were estimated from the previous year's General Ledger information + changes anticipated in those expenses and new expenses that might occur in the new year.

Take the first step in optimizing your practice.
Prepare a budget.

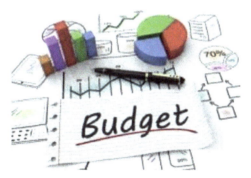

Remember, budgeting allows you to look at how you actually performed in a previous time period, it allows you to score yourself on how well you estimated revenue and expenses in the previous year, and it allows you to prepare a foundation for Forecasting (see next chapter).

An in depth explanation of how to prepare a Budget is beyond the scope of this book. If you would like help preparing a Budget, ask me about what we offer and how we can help you by emailing me at pjp@trackerenterprises.com.

*When it is obvious that
the goal cannot be reached,
don't adjust the goals;
adjust the action steps.*
Confucius

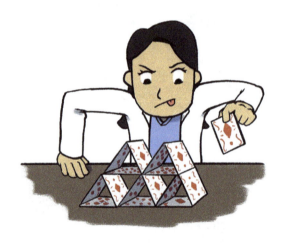

CHAPTER 19: FORECASTING - THE REAL GAME-CHANGER

Chance favors the prepared mind.[51]

You now understand that preparing annual budgets are necessary for laying the groundwork for all aspects of sound Business Life Cycle Management and planning. And you now know that a budget is a great starting point but only that – a starting point. After the budget has been prepared, however, **Forecasting** allows you to fine-tune the Optimal Business Management of your practice as changes occur.

While budgeting can be likened to looking in the rear view mirror, i.e., learning from what has occurred in the past, forecasting is like looking out the windshield to what is really happening in front of you in real time. *Obviously, you need both.*

Imagine how we learned to do things right as we matured. Human nature dictates that each of us must experience the consequences of our past actions before we can choose the path that works best in the future. *Wouldn't it be more advantageous to use information that historically proved valuable, and then adopt that knowledge to what is going on now and what might happen in the future?*

Therefore, we use financial forecasting as the foundation to move forward. By understanding the differences between budgeting and forecasting, planning the future by looking at the past and present might make the difference between the

> Don't allow luck to govern your future.

financial success and failure of your practice. After all, what good is it to plan on new facilities, equipment, staff, etc. if you have no idea what the financial burden will be based on what is currently happening in your business?

---

[51] Louis Pasteur

Forecasts take information prepared in the budget and then, they allow you to readjust your predicted numbers as actual new financial information is input. At best, budgets become historical information. Forecasts allow you to make necessary changes on a regular basis and are dependent on what is actually happening.

What exactly is a forecast?

To **Forecast** is to estimate, predict, or calculate, in advance, based on understanding historical information and planning for trends.[52] An example includes meteorologists' forecasts done on Monday for the next weekend; forecasts are updated as weather patterns change during the week with hopes of being as accurate as possible when the weekend arrives.

> When it comes to the future, history does not always repeat itself.

What's the difference between budgets and forecasts?

	Budgets	Forecasts
1	Done 1/year & then put aside as reference.	Usually done once per month
2	Planning the future by looking at the past.	Change as financial situation changes. Can do "what if" scenarios at any time.
3	Static and based on past performance.	Dynamic and change constantly.
4	Budgets are accounting-based.	Based on actual daily operations.
5	Budgets are the best way to plan for profits.	Adjust your plans to maximize profits.
6	Budgets leave profits to chance.	You have control over your profits.

Forecasting is the basis for planning

Forecasting should be the basis for your most important planning decisions. For example, you need to be able to predict how to plan for changes in scheduling, facility costs, labor requirements, inventory, production, purchasing, etc.

> Many things will change over the year; you must be able to react quickly.

---

[52] American Heritage Dictionary, 2016

Hierarchy of forecasting ...

As demonstrated in the last chapter, the Budget triangle is only balancing on one unstable point.

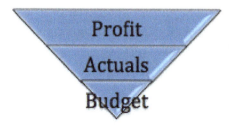

©Tracker Enterprises, Inc. 2018

After Actuals occur and new Forecasts are developed, the Budget is no longer what is managed to; it is now only a reference point. Every new Forecast becomes the basis to manage to.

Imagine, then, that the **Actuals** change values from the original Budget; then, every month, new bottom support triangles (**Forecasts**) are developed under the unstable **Budget** giving you more balance since you now know more about how the year is progressing. In this illustration, there are four **Forecast** triangles (e.g., four months of Actuals) below the original **Budget**. Each additional month of forecasting adds more stability and provides vital information needed to keep you on track.

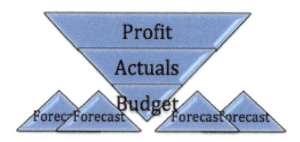

©Tracker Enterprises, Inc. 2018

Forecasting methodologies ...

Forecasting methods are divided into the following categories:

- **Qualitative Forecasting** is based on *subjective* opinion-based information gathering and interpretation.
- **Quantitative Forecasting** relies on implementing *objective* mathematical formulations.[53]

Qualitative Forecasting

The qualitative method is subjective, i.e., it uses judgment, experience, expertise, intuition, and opinions to arrive at forecasts. Qualitative forecasting is the most commonly used method. By studying your past financial history and then comparing those financials to the financials considered to be ideal for your healthcare profession, you can often predict, with a reasonable degree of accuracy, what the future year's and each month's revenue and expenses will be.

Quantitative Forecasting

Quantitative methods use mathematical and statistical techniques that make use of historical data accumulated over time. These methods assume that history repeats itself (i.e., what has occurred in the past will occur in the future). Variations of this method include studying moving averages that use demand in the past to predict demand in the future (e.g., if expenses increased last year by 5%, you might consider increasing the next year's by 5%).

By combining these methods, reliable predictions are possible.

> The best financial management method is the one that best fits the operating methods and optimal strategic plan *of your business*.

---

[53] Wikipedia. https://en.wikipedia.org/wiki/Forecasting

Reasons for forecasting ...

Because your existing and potential customers (i.e., patients) have the knowledge available, via media, the web, etc. to make educated decisions and then move rapidly from one source of service to another, you can never again allow yourself to look at your patients as stationary targets. Changes in customer loyalty may be due to any number of reasons, for example, cutting-edge technology, better customer service, competitive pricing, and/or (and most importantly) a perception of increased value for the money spent. It is essential that you consider how to forecast to stay ahead of the competition.

Forecasting allows you to combine insights with facts to make better decisions and *stops you from making emotional or gut decisions that may feel right at the time* but *don't hold water* after seeing the anticipated results after forecasting.

> If you manage the outcome of your business, *you must understand how to make a profit.*

Forecasting tools should provide you with an analysis of:

- **Production** needs to be watched since *small decreases in production might produce large decreases in revenue.*
- **Expenses** need to be watched since adjustments need to be made if revenue decreases or expenses increase.
- **Accounts receivables** need to be monitored for past due account balances. Some experts recommend that acceptable accounts receivable average 1½ times monthly production; this way, you have a cushion to fall back on as time passes. *I believe this is flawed since outstanding dollars really belong to you. Compensation must be in a timely fashion to cover costs. Your accounts receivable should only include dollars due from insurance and patients who have been put on payment plans.*
- **Inventory.** You need to know what products, that you carry in your office, are moving quickly and what products move slowly for purposes of smart ordering – *you want to provide rapid response to your patients' needs, but you don't want to stockpile and pay for items that rarely are used or sold.*

133

Inspect what you expect.

because

What gets measured
gets managed (done).
Peter Drucker

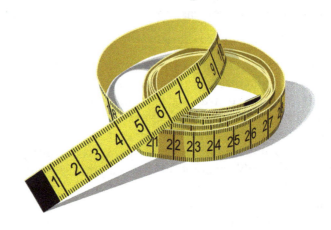

Sample Actuals & Forecasts ...

The Budget sample in Chapter 18 has been copied and now re-named as Actuals & Forecasts since it represents what is forecast for the year. This is what you would do at the beginning of the year. These samples are only summaries drawn from in-depth information found in our detailed accompanying spreadsheets.

FORECAST SUMMARY REPORT
DR. JOHN SAMPLE

FORECAST Summary	JAN FOR	FEB FOR	MAR FOR	APRIL FOR	MAY FOR	JUNE FOR	JULY FOR	AUG FOR	SEPT FOR	OCT FOR	NOV FOR	DEC FOR	YEAR FOR
PRODUCTION													
DOCTOR OWNER	100000	90000	100000	96000	100000	92000	96000	96000	92000	100000	90000	90000	1142000
DOCTOR ASSOCIATE	66800	61350	62150	65300	69050	59100	58250	63400	54900	70800	62500	57950	751550
PRODUCTS FOR RESALE	2213	2213	2213	2213	2213	2213	2213	2213	2213	2213	2213	2213	26556
TOTAL PRODUCTION	169013	153563	164363	163513	171263	153313	156463	161613	149113	173013	154713	150163	1920106
REVENUE													
SERVICES	143661	130529	139709	138986	145574	130316	132994	137371	126746	147061	131506	127639	1632090
MISC. INCOME OTHER	450	450	450	450	450	450	450	450	450	450	450	450	5400
ADJUSTMENTS TO INCOME	(836)	(836)	(836)	(836)	(836)	(836)	(836)	(836)	(836)	(836)	(836)	(836)	(10032)
TOTAL REVENUE	143275	130143	139323	138600	145188	129930	132608	136985	126360	146675	131120	127253	1627458
EXPENSES													
STAFF PAY & BENEFITS	49426	46112	56460	48631	47957	46173	44534	56146	43024	49158	45183	44172	576977
ASSOCIATE COMP	16700	15338	15538	16325	17263	14775	14563	15850	13725	17700	15625	14488	187888
CAPITAL & FACILITIES	6054	6750	8237	5754	6213	6204	6476	6204	8187	6104	4978	5254	76415
LAB	12000	12000	12000	12000	12000	12000	12000	12000	12000	12000	12000	12000	144000
SUPPLIES	16086	14321	14571	15931	14571	14316	16081	14316	14666	15831	14566	14316	179572
ADMINISTRATIVE	8700	5463	6823	6825	5463	6057	10266	5463	6923	9700	7463	6057	85202
MARKETING	6000	6000	6000	6000	6000	6000	6000	6000	6000	6000	6000	6000	72000
SUBTOTAL EXPENSES	114966	105983	119628	111466	109466	105525	109919	115979	104525	116493	105815	102287	1322053
TOTAL OP EXPENSES	96697	90146	103060	93572	91704	90169	93788	99629	89769	89836	88621	86768	1122759
TOTAL OP PROFIT	35751	2356	28150	40757	45447	34656	26830	35294	30898	46778	42935	33552	403404

In the sample Forecast (through April) below, actual values now appear in black; forecasted values stay blue.

FORECAST SUMMARY REPORT
ACTUALS /FORECASTS
DR. JOHN SAMPLE

FORECAST Summary	JAN ACT	FEB ACT	MAR ACT	APRIL ACT	MAY FOR	JUNE FOR	JULY FOR	AUG FOR	SEPT FOR	OCT FOR	NOV FOR	DEC FOR	YEAR FOR
PRODUCTION													
DOCTOR OWNER	104950	89700	103452	91756	100000	92000	96000	96000	92000	100000	90000	90000	1145858
DOCTOR ASSOCIATE	64725	68777	61616	64399	89050	59100	58250	63400	54900	70800	62500	57950	755467
PRODUCTS FOR RESALE	1875	2344	2155	1998	2213	2213	2213	2213	2213	2213	2213	2213	26076
TOTAL PRODUCTION	171550	160821	167223	158153	171263	153313	156463	161613	149113	173013	154713	150163	1927401
REVENUE													
SERVICES	106555	104343	138777	143011	145574	130316	132994	137371	126746	147061	131506	127639	1571892
MISC. INCOME OTHER	390	471	399	443	450	450	450	450	450	450	450	450	5303
ADJUSTMENTS TO INCOME	(951)	(454)	(799)	(811)	(836)	(836)	(836)	(836)	(836)	(836)	(836)	(836)	(9703)
TOTAL REVENUE	105994	104360	138377	142643	145188	129930	132608	136985	126360	146675	131120	127253	1567492
EXPENSES													
STAFF PAY & BENEFITS	53353	4711	55815	46887	47957	46173	44534	56146	43024	49158	45183	44172	537113
ASSOCIATE COMP	17778	16180	17194	15404	17263	14775	14563	15850	13725	17700	15625	14488	190544
CAPITAL & FACILITIES	6513	6750	8237	5754	6213	6204	6476	6204	8187	6104	4978	5254	76874
LAB	13554	11778	14411	11353	12000	12000	12000	12000	12000	12000	12000	12000	147096
SUPPLIES	17111	14555	14715	13844	14571	14316	16081	14316	14666	15831	14566	14316	178888
ADMINISTRATIVE	8353	5561	6767	7215	5463	6057	10266	5463	6923	9700	7463	6057	85287
MARKETING	6000	6000	6000	6000	6000	6000	6000	6000	6000	6000	6000	6000	72000
SUBTOTAL EXPENSES	122662	65535	123139	106457	109466	105525	109919	115979	104525	116493	105815	102287	1287802
TOTAL OP EXPENSES	97845	88134	102898	95334	91704	90169	93788	99629	89769	89836	88621	86768	1123495
TOTAL OP PROFIT	8149	16226	35479	47309	45447	34656	26830	35294	30898	46778	42935	33552	403553

Sample Written Analysis of Actuals and Forecasts ...

This is an abbreviated sample of a written analysis for April. Imagine receiving this on a monthly basis so that you can understand the health of your practice in less than one hour.

Smith Healthcare Group

Actual/Forecast Report

Production & Revenue – (Actuals through April)

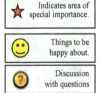

★	Indicates area of special importance.
☺	Things to be happy about.
❓	Discussion with questions

Production

 • Total doctors' Production was forecast at $210,100. Actual was $227,243 or $17,143 over forecast and $23,189 1more than last April.
  Doctors' production for the first 4 months was budgeted for $720,400. Actual was $748,321.

 • Total Other Providers' Production was forecast at $102,100. Actual was $106,289 or $4,189 more than forecast and $9,406 more than last April.
  Other' production for the first 4 months was budgeted for $418,800. Actual was $420,872.

 • Total Production was forecast at $312,200. Actual was $333,532 or $21,332 over forecast and $32,595 more than last April.
  Total production for the first 4 months was budgeted for $1,139,200. Actual was $1,169,893.
  This represents only a 3% decrease in Production for the first 4 months compared to last year.

Revenue

★ • The ratio of revenue to production was originally estimated at 74%. After the first 4 months, it is now re-estimated at 74%. We will follow this each month. This is still excellent for the large population of PPO & HMO patients that this practice has.

★ • Total Revenue was forecast at $227,906 and was budgeted at $232,952. Actual was $250,178 or $22,272 more than forecast and $17,226 more than budgeted. Total Revenue was $32,472 more than last April.
  Total Revenue for the first 4 months was budgeted for $843,008. Actual was $858,615.
  This represents only a 5% decrease in Revenue for the first 4 months compared to last year.

Accounts Receivable (A/R)

• Total A/R increased from $75,846 to $81,294.

• Current A/R over 90 days increased from $9,816 last month to $10,919, an increase of $1,102.

Practice Analysis Statistics

• Total Patients seen were 1,334 of which 14% were Old Medicare, 4% were New Medicare, 4% were Assurant, and 78% were Fee for Service or PPO. Therefore, 22% of patients seen came from capitation plans.

Team Salaries

- Total Team Expenses including additional expenses/benefits were forecast at $71,442. Actuals were $69,563 or $1,879 less than forecast.
  Total Team Expenses for first 4 months were budgeted for $295,209. Actuals were $269,855.

Office Supplies

- Office Supplies were forecast at $1,575. Actuals were $1,552 or $23 less than forecast.
  Total Office Supplies for the first 4 months were budgeted for $6,530. Actuals were $8,531.

Clinical Supplies

- Clinical Supplies were forecast at $8,518. Actuals were $7,045 or $1,473 less than forecast.
  Total Clinical Supplies for the first 4 months were budgeted for $56,539. Actuals were $38,421.

Capital & Facilities

- Capital & Facilities forecast at $13,272. Actuals were $13,604 or $332 more than forecast.
  Capital & Facilities for the first 4 months were budgeted for $60,423. Actuals were $53,933.

Administrative

- Total Admin was forecast at $11,851. Actuals were $9,215 or $2,637 less than forecast mainly due to surgery referral fees being less than expected.
  Total Admin for the first 4 months was budgeted for $40,780. Actual was $46,161.

Total Operational Expenses

- Operational Expenses forecast at $183,845. Actuals at $167,817 or $16,028 less than forecast.
  Total Operating Expenses for first 3 months budgeted at $717,826. Actuals were $654,256.

Total Operational Profit

- Operational Profit was forecast at $44,061. Actual was $82,360 or $38,299 more than forecast.
  Total Operating Profit for the first 4 months was budgeted for $125,182. Actual was $204,089.

Other income/Expenses

- After Loans, Total Expenses forecast at $201,196. Actuals at $84,463 or $116,733 less.
  Total Expenses for the first 4 months was budgeted for $818,620. Actual was $646,616.

Net Cash Flow

- Total Net Cash Flow was forecast at $26,710. Actual was $165,714 or $139,004 more than forecast. Year-end Net Cash Flow is now forecast at $306,166. *Total Net Cash Flow for the first 4 months was budgeted for $24,388. Actual was $212,000.*

Make forecasting a habit; you won't regret it.

We are what we repeatedly do.
Excellence, then, is not an act, but a habit.
Aristotle

> An in depth explanation of how to prepare a Forecast and how to Reforecast are beyond the scope of this book. If you would like help preparing a Forecast, ask me about what we offer and how we can help you by emailing me at pjp@trackerenterprises.com.

SECTION IV: SUMMARY & OPTIMIZE ACTION PLAN

Optimize Summary:

1. Key functions of Optimal Business Management in your practice:
   a. Maintaining and understanding your bookkeeping system
   b. Information tools including ways to monitor, measure, and manage using Key Performance Indicators (KPIs)
2. Regardless of your choice, you need to become versed in business
   a. If you are planning on the military, you will enter into private or corporate practice after the military.
   b. If you work as an employee, you need to understand business so that you can negotiate for what you are worth.
   c. If you are in a specialty program, you will, at some point, be going into private practice or working as an employee.
3. Questions to continually ask yourself:
   a. Is the practice experiencing unusual gains or losses?
   b. Are profits holding or improving?
   c. Are profits keeping pace with expenses?
   d. How does cash flow compare with profit?
   e. Are changes consistent with the growth needed?
   f. Are there any signs of financial distress?
   g. Are there any unusual assets and liabilities?
4. Why is a Budget necessary and how to prepare it?
5. Why are Forecasts necessary and how to prepare them?
6. What you measure is what you get. So, remember to
   a. Set up your KPIs (Key Performance Indicators)
   b. Test everything and retest every month
   c. Measure the results and find tune the process every month

Optimize Action Plan: The Road Map

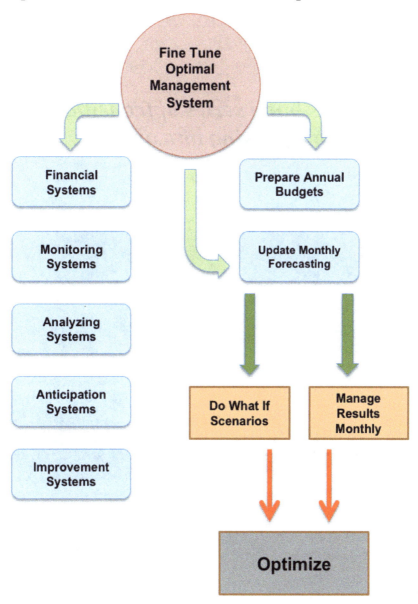

©Tracker Enterprises, Inc.

Life is but a series of transitions,
one passing into another.

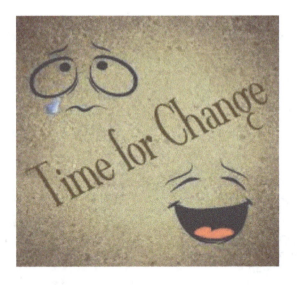

Section V: Sell

Chapter 20: My Story Continues With a Surprise

I am convinced that life is 10% what happens to me
and 90% of how I react to it.
Charles Swindoll

After twenty-five years of a very successful practice, my life was permanently altered by a medical disability. OOPS!!! I had ignorantly believed that I had at least 10-15 more years left in making my practice and myself more successful. Now, the money stopped pouring in, and I was forced to re-visit my naivety of business in relation to transition planning; I had not prepared a game plan for such an early exit from my practice.

After the sale of my practice, I tried retirement for one year. I had spent my life serving and being around people; I was lonely and retirement lacked the mental and social stimulation I had been accustomed to. Retirement surely didn't work for me.

My daughter came to my rescue. She made me aware of the new life paradigm: *"Everyone should plan to pursue numerous careers throughout his/her life."* She gave me this quote to ponder:

What is the end of life to the caterpillar
is the beginning of life to the butterfly.
Lao Tzu (paraphrased)

I found that other healthcare professionals, regardless of their chosen professions and number of years in practice, were experiencing transition dilemmas with having very little, if any, knowledge of exit planning. These doctors had been deluded into thinking that they could practice as long as they wanted and then, when they were ready to exit, someone would automatically appear ready to buy their practices at the price the exiting doctor expected. On top of that, many of them continued to slow down as they got older with subsequent decreases in annual revenues and therefore, decreases in the practice values. Those exiting doctors had misunderstood that buyers don't want to pay for a practice the way it was ten years ago; they pay for today's value.

Since I no longer had the ability to provide clinical care and I was ill prepared regarding exit planning, I became determined that other healthcare professionals should not have to experience what I did.

A philosophy and program were developed to allow healthcare professionals to understand, regardless of which life cycle their business was in, to do "exit planning" well in advance of when they originally expected to transition out of their practices. This exit planning road map included the absolute necessity of being prepared to exit from Day 1, just in case the practitioner experienced a catastrophic reason to leave practice whether that reason 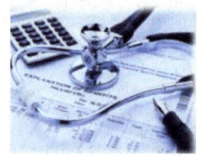 occurred shortly after starting the practice or after forty years of practice or anytime in between. The plan also included how to value the practice at any time in the Business Life Cycle or when an exit was being anticipated.

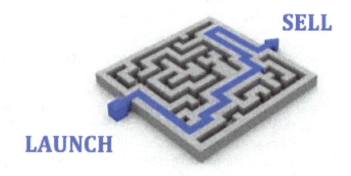

Chapter 21: You - Prepare an End Game Plan

Planning is bringing the future into the present
so that you can do something about it now.
Alan Lakein

When to prepare an Exit Plan

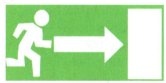

Planning an exit can seem like a daunting task involving a lot of time – time that you don't have. In addition, several issues need to be considered including building the value of your practice so that you can exit at the selling price you want and deciding on what you want to do with your life after you leave.

Remember that I said earlier in the book that you have to be prepared at any time and at all times. As I mentioned previously about the importance of preparing a written Business Plan from the get go, preparing a written Exit Plan is also essential. *Most of us would never consider not having a Will prepared in advance.*

A common Exit Planning paradox is that most doctors don't want to give up control of their practices before they're ready, but they also don't want to spend much time on Exit Planning. Having an Exit Plan gives you a chance to maintain control of the process.

How to start preparing an Exit Plan …

A real benefit in preparing a <u>written</u> Exit Plan is that it can increase your chance for success. Written goals are more likely to be executed than verbal goals. Additionally, written Exit Plans encourage accountability and are clearer and more specific than verbal communication. The act of writing causes business owners to think more carefully, which decreases chances for future misinterpretation. *Consider that individuals are 42% more likely to achieve their goals just by writing them down.*[54]

---

[54] Matthews, Gail. Psychology professor at Dominican University, California.

In a written Exit Plan, all advisors are assigned specific responsibilities and deadlines; i.e., it helps everyone involved avoid procrastination and keeps everyone, especially you, accountable. Having a Plan with built-in deadlines and responsibilities will help you to avoid falling prey to the "rolling five-year plan," wherein you're always looking to exit five years from now.

> I had one client in the northeastern U.S. who I coached for over 15 years. Every year, during our budget planning meetings, I asked him when he might want to retire. Every year, for 10 years, he told me: "*I think I'd like to call it quits in about five years.*"

With a written plan, you can maintain control of your practice until you're ready to give it up, and you don't have to make Exit Planning your primary focus. This can increase your planning efficiency and give you the time to continue to build your practice's value.

How long should Exit Planning take?

In general, creating an Exit Plan can take several weeks to months, while executing the Plan can take several years – another good reason to start NOW. Creating and executing an Exit Plan usually requires input from owners and several advisors and should also involve an owner's family and management team.

Do Exit Plans evolve?

"Written down" does not translate to "chiseled in stone." Like I indicated previously about how Business Plans should be reworked as time passes, written Exit Plans can, and often do, change. As your practice and goals evolve, updating an Exit Plan gives your planning strategies credibility as time passes.[55]

---

[55] Stiefler, Ken. *The Exit Planning Review*. July 2018.

When is the best time to sell?

Since I had personally experienced a career-ending disability, without prior warning, I am very familiar with why an owner needs to be prepared to sell at any time. I emphasize again, plan for this in advance, no matter what stage of development your business life cycle is in, whether you are:

1. Preparing to start a practice (**Launch**),
2. Enhancing or restructuring your practice (**Expand**),
3. Fine tuning a practice (**Optimize**),
4. Considering retirement or exit (**Sell**).

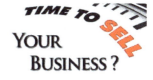

This exit planning includes:

- Anyone interested in selling in the near or distant future.
- Anyone who has a need to know the value of a practice for reasons such as preparing a business plan, requesting a bank loan, or anyone wanting to buy a practice.
- Anyone wanting to improve the value drivers.
- Anyone wanting to monitor, measure, evaluate, and then, adjust operations so that the business increases in value.

Don't wait until you have to sell; start preparing now. You will need a map before you go into the woods. Let's start looking at what you need to know and how to prepare that map so you are ready. – AT ANY TIME!

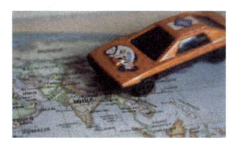

I found that healthcare professionals, regardless of their chosen professions and number of years in practice, were experiencing dilemmas caused by having little, if any, knowledge of their finances and how that might relate to a future transition out of their practices. These practice owners had been deluded by their educators, mentors and peers into thinking that other advisors (accountants, attorneys, consultants, etc.) would offset any need to understand finance and exit strategies. The bottom line is - your knowledge (not someone else's) is what counts.

> *Someone is sitting in the shade today because someone planted a tree a long time ago.*
> Warren Buffett

Are you really in touch with your future?

Face it - like every business owner, you will one day exit your practice either voluntarily or involuntarily. On that day you will want to have met certain business and personal objectives: the first (and usually prerequisite to all others) is financial security.

Believe it or not, most practice owners do absolutely nothing to plan. It is estimated that 80-86% of all small business owners have made no advance preparations; therefore, only 14-20% of current business owners have done exit strategy preparations.

Do you have a plan?

To avoid planning not only puts your future financial security at risk, it overlooks your practice's need to grow in value. Growing and protecting value is at the core of your exit planning strategies.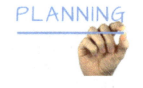

It makes sense to start planning for your eventual exit because you have to plan, measure, monitor, evaluate, implement and improve if you ever want to exit with the goals you have established. The simple reality is that most owners don't plan, and therefore, most owners are never able to leave their practices as they had dreamed of doing.

What are some exit planning excuses?

The three most common excuses owners use to justify delaying and or ignoring exit planning are:

1. The practice isn't worth enough to meet my financial needs yet. When it is, I'll start to think about how to exit (sell).
2. I don't need to plan. When I'm ready, a buyer will find me.
3. I can't imagine my life without my practice: I'll just keep working until I can't work anymore.

Let's examine these excuses.

Excuse #1: The practice is not worth enough at this time.

Why spend time, effort and money to plan an exit when today, you can't? Why not wait until it is theoretically possible to leave before beginning the exit planning? Here's why: unexpected things happen, e.g., divorce, a career-ending disability, death, etc. From Day 1, don't miss the opportunity to plan:

- Establish your personal exit goals and objectives.
- Based on the goals, prepare an exit plan that identifies the most productive actions you can take to create and protect value and to do so in the most tax-efficient way possible.
- Drive up your practice's value to the point where you can sell and exit with the cash necessary to achieve financial security.

Growing value usually does not occur unless owners focus their efforts on deliberate actions that move their practices toward their goals. These actions include continuing to add value drivers (more on value drivers later, but this will introduce you to the concept) to your practice that will result in it being worth more. Examples include:

- Improving your customer (patient) base,
- Keeping your equipment current and in good working order,
- Building a strong employee base,
- Keeping accounts receivables collectible and to a minimum,
- Developing a strong management team,
- Having a powerful marketing program, etc.

Excuse #2: There will always be good buyers for practices.

Buyers don't grow on trees; you have to cultivate them. This can be accomplished by developing a relationship with local healthcare education facilities, military institutions, associateship bases of operation, practice transition experts, practice brokers, supply representatives familiar with practices and buyers in your area, etc. so that you can make them aware of your existence (read *Where can you find potential buyers* later in this chapter).

Excuse #3: I love practicing. I'll practice until I can't.

The answers to the other two excuses above relate directly to the question: "*Who knows when and why that will be?*" You may have some idea when you want to exit or you may simply want to practice the rest of your life -- that's fine, as long as you have the physical and mental capacity to do so. However, as you saw in my case, things happen – ALWAYS at the most unexpected times.

Is exit planning worth it?

> **Before any beginning,**
> **there needs to be a plan of**
> **how you are going to get to the end.**
> Byron Pulsifer

You need to begin to think in terms of your personal and financial goals well in advance. Since tackling a task of this magnitude can be daunting, practice owners often ask whether devoting the time and money to a project of this magnitude is really worth the effort. The complexity of transition planning can be significant since it includes issues such as a practice valuation, taxation, legal documentation, financial planning and especially the emotional aspects associated with planning for the exiting process and not knowing what you will do next in your life. It is imperative that you understand that good planning can be the difference between a successful transition and a complete collapse of all your goals. The emphasis needs to be on "Planning," which will then support the "Exiting" process.

When should you start exit planning?

The correct answer is "yesterday." But, you need to start sometime and now (today) is the best answer.

It doesn't matter whether you have just started your practice (e.g., going from school to ownership, going from associateship/employee to ownership, going from military service to ownership, etc.), whether you have been in business for one year or thirty years, or whether you are planning to retire in the near future, <u>you need to have a plan now</u>!

Will there be a market for your practice?

If you plan to sell, you will want to attract the largest market of potential buyers. **If you are a buyer**, you will want to choose from as many practices as you can find. In order to do so, you need to understand market conditions.

- **Seller/Purchaser Ratios** – There is always an imbalance in the ratio of sellers and purchasers. Currently, there are fewer purchasers than sellers mainly due to the large numbers of baby boomers approaching retirement and wanting to exit their practices. In addition, many healthcare professional schools have decreased class sizes and some have closed.
- **Demographic Factors** - There is currently an increased interest in practicing in urban environments with many small town or rural areas finding it difficult to attract healthcare professionals. In other words, the chances of making an excellent living may be more likely in a city environment than in less populated locales.
- **Increased Planning Time Frames** – The old philosophy of deciding to leave a practice with a year or less planning is gone. Now, the ideal is planning well in advance.
- **Marketing the Opportunity** – With more sellers than buyers available, the need for marketing becomes more evident. Current owners will need to differentiate their practices to make them more attractive to potential buyers. This requires planning and may result in the need to improve the office appearance, to update the equipment, etc.

What else should you consider?

Owners (and their families) who wait until the last minute to decide how much cash they want and need from their practices do so emotionally and reactively. They often make hasty decisions or are blinded by attractive "offers" held out by unscrupulous buyers. If an owner has one foot out the door, finding out the practice is not worth what he or she had hoped can be a painful and expensive experience. Even more painful is the subsequent rededication of efforts needed in trying to re-build the value of the practice. Owners often don't realize that focused attention on growing value is an essential part of the exit. Why not do this now instead of waiting for the inevitable?

PLAN
PLAN
PLAN
PLAN
ACTION

It's not uncommon, nor is it abnormal, for owner/doctors to want to slow down as the years in practice go by. Here's something else to watch out for, though. As I said earlier, if you start cutting back days and hours you work each week, and if you take longer vacations as the years go by, you will realize less production and revenue and therefore, less profitability. Potential buyers will not want to pay for the value you had in previous years when you were more productive; they want to pay for what the practice is producing right now. This can be avoided by bringing in doctor employees and other ancillary producers who can bring the revenue back to what it was or better. Remember, however, that you may earn less personally, and labor expenses will increase. The moral of the story is, you can slow down, but don't let your practice slow down.

Another reality -- life happens: An example is a close friend who owned a very large and profitable group practice in another city. He was at the top of his game. A few days before his 60th birthday, he passed away suddenly and without prior warning. His family was immediately tasked with what to do and had no idea what the practice was worth. Don't let this happen to you. With guidance, they realized a sales price 400% higher than what they originally guessed the practice was worth. Remember, however, the value of a practice falls rapidly when the senior doctor suddenly is unable to service his/her patients.

Start with the end in mind

Understand your objectives. Get involved methodically and proactively. On an annual basis, do a summary valuation of your practice. Pretend you are getting ready to sell your business in the next twelve months. Some good questions you should start asking include:

- Who will be your advisors (e.g., attorneys, accountants, transition facilitators, brokers, potential buyers)?
- How will you go about valuing the practice?
- What goals will you need to meet for your financial future?
- How will you settle accounts receivables and payables?
- How will existing bank loans, etc. be paid off?
- How will equipment and building leases be settled?
- How will employees and patients be notified, etc., etc.?

By utilizing an organized and systematic Exit Planning process, owners can place a realistic value on their practices.[56] Always remember this:

Every entrepreneur should build his company with an eye toward eventually selling it, regardless of the exit strategy. When you build to sell, you learn to look at your business the way a potential buyer would look at it.[57]

Protect yourself and your family

At this stage, you've already done what it takes to make your practice successful. You hired the right people, provided excellent service, and developed high-quality relationships with your patients. You did all of this by careful planning and executing. The same process that applied to starting and running a successful practice applies to any successful business exit.

---

[56] Stiefler, Ken. *The Exit Planning Review*. Business Enterprises Institute. 2016.

[57] Brodsky, Norm. INC Magazine. June 2013.

Whether you're looking to exit your practice in 10 months, 10 years, etc., one fact governs them all: <u>all owners, even the hardest working most dedicated workaholics, will exit their practices someday whether by choice, death, or otherwise</u>. You need to be able to answer the question, *"What will happen to me, my practice, and my family upon my exit?"* The consequences of proper planning have real effects on the things you care about most.

This is a summary of the exit strategy we discussed so far:

1. **Establish Goals:** Establish one foundational goal - exiting with financial security. Then establish secondary goals such as an exit date, successor, and getting the money you want.
2. **Measure, monitor and evaluate:** Start by knowing where you are today. Establish your practice's value. This will tell you whether you will have the money you need from the sale to exit with financial security at any point in your life cycle.
3. **Maximize and Protect Business Value:** Focus on growing and protecting your practice's value to give yourself the best chance to leave your practice when you want and for the money you need. Remember that revenue increases do not necessarily make the practice worth more (i.e., you added more expenses, loans, etc.); what is important is that the profitability continues to increase.
4. **Create your team:** You will need to prepare yourself well in advance of the sale. Don't delay in creating an experienced team and making sure your practice is the one that the greatest number of buyers will want to acquire.
5. **Ensure business continuity:** Protect your family and business if you die (e.g., an adequate life insurance policy for yourself and a key man policy for your practice) or become permanently incapacitated (e.g., a disability policy preferably paid by you personally to eliminate taxation). Your primary goal should be to give your family, employees, and customers the peace of mind that they will be protected and taken care of if something happens to you. This means having a strong staff foundation, continuing to grow the practice, having solid management, and making sure the programs are in place to allow your practice to continue to grow with or without you.

Where can you find potential buyers?

- **Direct mail** – If you already have specific potential buyers' contact information, send a personalized letter. (If you want to grab a potential buyer's attention, write them a personal letter – no one does this anymore.) Target groups include:

  BUYERS GUIDE

  - Associates who are already employed by someone else.
  - Military doctors have already gained clinical experience.
  - Healthcare schools often have eager potential buyers.
- **Networking** – A great and inexpensive way to look for potential buyers. Put your information on your website, Facebook, LinkedIn (especially good for recruiting).
- **Consultants and Brokers** – These usually already have a list of potential buyers. Fees may include one or combination of:
  - A flat fee: usually collected up front, including all of the structuring (valuation, cash flow projections, financing, employment agreements, sales documents, etc.).
  - A flat fee: usually collected up front <u>but not including</u> the marketing; this will be done by you at your cost.
  - A commission of, on average, 10% of the sales price.
- **Supply Company Representatives** – Check with your supply reps. They are loyal to you and want to help. They typically have a list of potential buyers. Also, many major supply companies have in-house brokerage services.
- **Healthcare schools** – Most universities now have placement departments to assist upcoming graduates.
- **Print media** – Classified ads in professional journals can be very effective but are often very expensive.[58]

Why setting goals is important, even if they change

Having the foresight to set actionable goals combined with the flexibility to change them when necessary gives you the freedom to pursue your vision of a successful exit. Let's look at three

---

[58] Hill, Roger K. *Transitions*. ADA. 2006.

reasons why setting goals is so important, even though those goals might change.

1. **Establishes Your Target**: Goal setting allows you to establish a target that defines what a successful exit looks like for you, your family, and your practice. These goals can help prepare for the selling process and get you on the path toward success.

2. **Provides a Road Map**: Setting goals helps you develop a road map for how to achieve your goals and confidence to properly prepare for the journey. Setting goals also helps you track where you are on your journey toward Exit Planning success. Having an appreciation for where you are on the path toward your exit goals can encourage you to stay the course when times are good and refocus and reevaluate if things aren't going as planned.

3. **Addresses Conflicts Before They Do Damage**: Establish your foundational goals:
   a. Exiting with financial security
   b. Exiting when you choose
   c. Exiting for the money you want
   d. Transferring the business to whom you choose
   e. Keeping your legacy alive
   f. Keeping your staff employed with benefits[59]

REMEMBER

Hope is not an effective business strategy. [60]

---

[59] Stiefler, Ken. *The Exit Planning Review*. Business Enterprises Institute. 2016.

[60] Smith, Mark S. A., From MSP to BSP, pre release, 2018

CHAPTER 22: INTRODUCTION TO THE VALUATION

A fundamental aspect of a successful business exit is assuring that your practice has enough value to allow you to exit with financial security. This, along with the value of your assets, gives you the best chance to pursue the exit you want on the timeline you want. Obtaining a proper, professional practice valuation is the first step in determining how much your practice is worth.

What you should initially provide to a potential buyer?

The Practice Valuation is your presentation of what the practice is worth. It is often called "The Book" or "The Offering." This is where you put your best foot forward and explain everything a potential buyer may want to know about your practice.

It is where you tell the buyer:

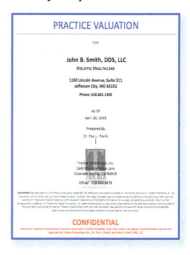

- What you desire the transaction to be
- Differentiating qualities of your practice
- Competitive advantages (e.g., location, equipment, services)
- Growth opportunities
- Profitability existing and potential
- All other value drivers defined and quantified

A comprehensive valuation should contain the following:

- Executive Summary
- Industry analysis & outlook
- Business overview/history
- Organization structure (e.g., corporate structure, etc.)
- Practice characteristics
- Operating income analysis

- Adjusted earning projections
- Tangible assets
- Description of products, services, processes, etc.
- Description of staff positions but not names
- Define the valuation process & show valuation calculations
- Current Fair Market Value
- Sales, marketing & growth opportunities
- Competitive landscape, risks and limitations
- Financial discussion (Balance sheets, P&Ls, forecasts, etc.)
- Photographs of exterior and interior
- Map showing location of office(s)
- Information including owner's discretionary expenses

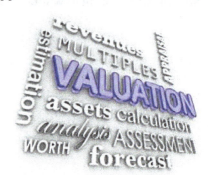

The practice valuation generally should also include ...

1. Purpose of the valuation
2. Assumptions
3. Economic analysis (a.k.a., the Beige Book)
4. Practice characteristics
5. Revenue vs. production comparisons
6. Introduction to the valuation process
7. Valuation methods used
8. Advantages of the practice
9. Important notes to consider
10. Practice valuation questionnaire
11. Photos of surrounding areas
12. Qualifications of the evaluator
13. Disclaimer

How to arrive at a value for the practice ...

The fair market value (price) of a healthcare practice is an estimate of the market value of a business based on what a knowledgeable, willing, and unpressured buyer would pay to a knowledgeable, willing, and unpressured seller. Fair market value differs from intrinsic value (the value placed on an asset based on owner's or seller's preferences and circumstances).[61]

The valuation is a process and set of procedures used to determine the practice's worth. There are many methods used to determine what a practice is worth. Value means different things to different sellers, buyers and evaluators. For example, an owner may believe the practice "blue sky" (intrinsic value based on the practice's connection to its patient base) is worth a considerable amount; a buyer, however, may think that the fair market value should be entirely determined by its historic income and future income potential. Therefore, a final evaluation of the practice's market value may be determined by a number of methods or averaging of those methods.[62]

The five steps typically used to value a practice typically include:

1. **Planning**: The owner plans to sell the practice to the highest and most suited bidder. This step introduces why the practice is unique in the marketplace and why the price is justified.

2. **Preparing the financial statements**: To do a proper job of valuing a practice, three years of historic income statements, balance sheets, and tax returns are typically used.

3. **Choosing the valuation methods**: Most valuation methods are in the form of one or more of the following approaches:

    a. Asset approach: This focuses on a business's net asset value (NAV), or the fair-market value (FMV), of its total assets minus its total liabilities to determine what it would cost to re-create the business.

---

[61] Wikipedia. https://en.wikipedia.org/wiki/Fair_market_value

[62] Sletten, Paul. The Sletten Group. Denver, CO. Many thanks for your mentorship.

b. Market approach: An apples-to-apples comparison (similar to doing comps in the housing real estate market) might be difficult to gather because sufficient meaningful comparison data might be unavailable. Most practices do not often lend themselves to a market comparison approach.

c. Income approach: This method determines worth based on earning potential and is usually considered the most accurate. Income-based methods rely on taking the net operating income (NOI) and dividing it by the capitalization (CAP) rate.

4. **Applying selected valuation methods**: Since calculating practice values should produce justifiable results, several methods should be used to crosscheck assumptions.

5. **Reaching the practice value conclusion**: After all of the above is considered, the actual practice worth can be estimated. Since the various methods chosen may produce somewhat different results, concluding the value requires that these differences be reconciled to derive the business value conclusion. Therefore, an average of the different valuation methods should be used in reaching the value.

Valuation methods typically used ...

This describes the methods used to estimate a range for the fair market value of the practice. This concept assumes that a practice is being valued as a viable operating entity and one that has its assets and inventory in place, its work force in place, and its doors open for business with no visible threat of discontinuance as a going business. The current methods (in order of most accurate being first, etc.) used for valuing a practice include:

1. **Discounted Cash Flow Method**: This is usually the most mathematically precise of the valuation methods. The idea is to appraise the practice value based on the expected future benefits that the buyer expects after purchase. The question answered is: If you buy the business today for a certain amount of money, receive annual cash flows over the period

you own the business, then sell the business, what return on your initial purchase investment do you get? Also, is the return on investment commensurable with the risk of owning the business compared to an alternative safe investment?

2. **Capitalized (CAP) Excess Earnings Method**: This approach is especially well suited for the valuation of practices with a stable predictable earnings history. If the practice shows steady profits year to year, the CAP method is a good choice. This approach assumes a practice is valued as a sum equaling the total of the tangible and intangible assets (including "goodwill"). Goodwill represents the amount of money a buyer would pay over the fair value of the Tangible Assets to acquire a practice that is well established and has a significant patient base thus assuring an assumed stabile monthly income. The value of a successful business generally exceeds the value of its assets since it takes time, effort and resources to make a business successful.

3. **Multiple of Discretionary Earnings Method**: This calculates the earnings track record and future prospects, likelihood of business and industry growth, business location, employee skill and stability, how attractive the business will, and how attractive the business financing or purchase terms are.[63]

Valuation criteria to consider ...

Valuation considerations are also based on the following criteria:

- The history of the practice and the types of services provided
- Training, education and experience of the doctor/owner
- Trends in the economy in the area served by this practice
- The size and growth rate of this practice
- Practice development, client flow, and case acceptance
- The effectiveness of the management of the practice
- Training, education, experience, and dedication of the team and the potential for retaining their services

---

[63] Sletten, Paul. The Sletten Group. Denver, CO.

Minimum items needed to evaluate a practice ...

1. Financial statements prepared by owner's accountant by year for the last two complete years and for current year-to-date.

2. List of personal expenses that would not be part of the business on a go-forward basis (vehicles, family salaries, donations, continuing education, etc.)

3. Practice Operating Data

   a. Total patient visits by month for the past 24 months
   b. New patient visits by month for the past 24 months
   c. Production by procedure codes
   d. Operating days and hours of practice
   e. Production by all providers for the past two years
   f. List of participating PPOs and HMOs (capitation)

4. Facility, e.g., lease terms, square footage, and renewal options

5. Description of marketing programs used

Detailed valuation items you will want to know ...

1. General Information
   a. Practice name, address and phone number
   b. How long has the practice been established
   c. Business structure (proprietor, S-Corp, LLC, C-Corp)
   d. Operating hours and number of days worked in the last two years
   e. Does the practice have other locations
   f. Is the current owner willing to stay on after the sale
   g. Any malpractice claims in the last 5 years
   h. Is the owner willing to provide any or all financing
2. Operational Information
   a. How many weeks ahead is each provider scheduled
   b. What procedures/treatments are unique to this office
   c. Is a computer system used and what is software used
3. Community Factors
   a. How would the area around the office be described (e.g., suburban, urban, rural, commercial, residential)

    b. What type of thoroughfare is the office located on (e.g., 2-lane street, 4-lane street, etc.) & accessibility

    c. Patient parking (e.g., free, paid, garage, street, etc.)

    d. Number of like practices within a 3 mile radius

    e. Is the population growing, stable or declining

4. Facility Factors

    a. Square footage of office

    b. Number of treatment rooms and other rooms

    c. Practice location (e.g., professional building, general office building, strip mall, major shopping mall, etc.)

    d. Is the office space owned, rented, shared, etc.

    e. If the owner owns the space, is rent paid to the owner

    f. If leased, what is remaining time: is lease renewable

    g. What does the rent include (e.g., utilities, etc.)

5. Patient Information

    a. Number of total patients seen in the last 2 years

    b. New patients seen per month for last 2 years

    c. Sources patients come from (e.g., patient referrals, yellow pages, website, Facebook, etc.)

    d. What clinical procedures are referred out

6. What was the total accounts receivables last month

Current   30 – 60 days   61 – 90 days   Over 91 days   Total

7. Staff Information

    a. Staff salaries, hours worked, etc.

    b. How many staff are employed and in what positions

8. Recent pictures of the outside and inside of the office

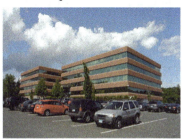 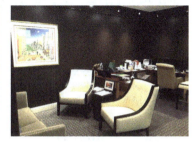

CHAPTER 23: HOW TO INCREASE PRACTICE VALUE

What happens if your practice isn't worth enough to allow you to exit with financial security? How can you increase your practice's value if everything that's made it successful thus far isn't enough? The answer lies in managing to the **Value Drivers**.

What Are Value Drivers?

Value Drivers are specific characteristics that drive growth. The following areas will have the greatest impact on your practice's value.

1. **Transferability**: Will a transfer of ownership be seamless and can it run independently of the current owner?
2. **Operating systems**: Are systems in place that will allow for increased cash flow?
3. **Demonstrated scalability**: Are the physical plant and staff prepared for and accepting to changes in hours, days, etc.?
4. **Diversified customer base**: Do patients come from varied bases (age, families, locations, insurance carriers, etc.) or are they limited to one or only a few sources?
5. **Proven growth strategy**: Does the practice show growth year in and year out? Do you have plans in place for growth?
6. **Is revenue sustainable**: Is current revenue sustainable? Are plans in place to replace revenue if the patient base changes?
1. **Size of office**: Is the entire space producing revenue?
2. **Location**(s): Is it in a safe, prosperous, area that attracts the clientele you will want?
3. **Management**: Is management staff complete and trained?
4. **Growth rate**: Is the profitability increasing each year?
5. **Employee mix**: Are there too many or too few employees? Is the mix of job descriptions producing maximum revenue?
6. **Diversified patient base**: Is the patient mix strong enough that if one segment leaves, the impact will be minimal?
7. **Vendor relationships**: Do you have a good or adversarial relationship with your vendors?
8. **Geographic coverage**: Do patients come from only nearby areas or do you attract patients from a large radius?

Why Value Drivers Matter

Growing practice value and cash flow can help you add to what your practice is currently worth. Potential buyers will look at:

- **Value Drivers**: historical cash-flow, sales growth, growth opportunities, market share, profitability, unique services, key employees, transferable, good systems, leadership, good financials so buyer can obtain financing.
- **Value Killers**: inconsistent profit, bad financials, poor management, no growth opportunity, and owner skills and patients who are not transferable.

> CONCERN: Untimely disclosure of the Seller's intent to employees, patients, vendors, and the marketplace could all potentially have negative impacts on the value of the business and the ability to sell it.

Benefits of Value Drivers:

- **Perspective**. Identifying and enhancing Value Drivers can help you view your business through the eyes of a prospective buyer. This helps you overcome sentimental attachments to your practice and decisions that only benefit you personally.
- **Action**. Because you've already set your goals and determined how much your business is worth, you know how much and how quickly growth needs to occur. This gives you an action plan.
- **Triage.** By identifying Value Drivers, you can concentrate your and your staff's efforts on areas that need the greatest improvement.[64]

---

[64] Stiefler, Ken. *The Exit Planning Review*. Business Enterprises Institute. 2016.

Business models for exit strategy planning

Even though you may be no where near ready to sell your practice, a great way to prepare your practice to run at its maximum potential is to model it to sell for as much as possible and to meet all three of the following requirements needed if you were to sell your practice. Obviously, you will want to sell it for as much as possible, but you may want to think of it this way.

- **Immediate Sale**: Pretend that you *will need* to sell your practice *tomorrow*. (Everything must be in place to value the practice).

- **Immediate Financing**: Pretend that you *will need* to obtain major financing *tomorrow*. (Everything must be in order before seeking out a potential lender).

- **Franchising**: Pretend that you *will need* to sell your business model as a franchise *tomorrow*. (Franchises are usually modeled after an ideal business road map. Think of your practice this way).

Immediate Sale

Start with the philosophy of having an end in mind. Work toward the goal of having your practice always prepared to sell, at the highest price, to the biggest audience, at any time – <u>all of the time</u>.

Therefore, even if you are just starting in your practice, begin by visualizing what the final goal of your business will be – *selling it*. Ask yourself the following questions (by the way, you should ask these same questions if you want to purchase a practice):

- *How much* will you want for it?
- *When* will you want to sell it?
- *Will there be* enough buyers?
- If you had to sell tomorrow, **would you get** what you want?
- If you sold tomorrow, **would the buyer get what the buyer wants**?

> To sell your business at any time, have it *always* ready to sell **right now**.

Immediate Financing

Every practice owner should always assume that his/her practice is in desperate need of a loan (just in case). Today, lending institutions prefer that you come to the table with a Business Plan before they lend you money. If you prepare a well-defined plan, and if you update your plan as time passes, lenders will see that you have an excellent business mind with the foresight to dynamically make adjustments when needed so that you can reach your predetermined goals via the shortest path and in the least amount of time. If the plan is viable, the loan process is significantly simplified.

Once you grasp the importance of the plan, you will understand that it serves the two purposes mentioned:

1. It serves as your road map, and
2. If you do need funding in the future, all of the information will be in place, at any given time, for the lending institutions.

Franchising

One more thought on the importance of planning - why do you think the general business world franchise model has a greater success rate when compared to the independent business models? Franchises typically report a 95% success rate in contrast to a 50% for independents. Franchises succeed because the model has been thoroughly researched and a system has been put in place to succeed. Even though healthcare practices do not typically lend themselves to franchising, the success model still works.

An in depth explanation of how to prepare a Practice Valuation is beyond the scope of this book. If you would like help preparing a Valuation, ask me about what we offer and how we can help you by emailing me at pjp@trackerenterprises.com.

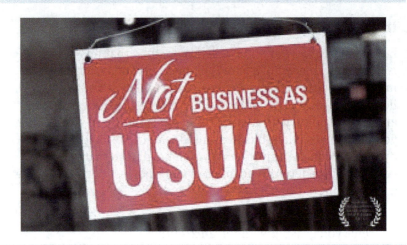

CHAPTER 24: SHOULD YOU CONSIDER AN HSO?

While your practice is extremely important, you should be able to maintain some semblance of work-life balance. If managing your business is taking over to the point where you're not prioritizing self-care and patient care, then you will need to reevaluate because if you let it get too far, you may experience burnout.

If you are thinking about selling your practice but wondering what you will do next, this may interest you. Let's assume that you still like practicing and treating patients, and you want some alternative other than completely leaving the healthcare profession. Maybe, however,

1. You want money now, not later, for whatever reason.
2. You are tired of the headaches involved in managing the business end of your practice; you simply want to treat patients, and that's it.

A fairly recent alternative to selling or changing ownership of a practice is to consider Healthcare Service Organizations (HSOs). Healthcare Service Organizations, also known in the industry as "Healthcare Support Organizations" are independent business support centers that contract with healthcare practices. They provide critical business management and support, including non-clinical operations.

Support services provided by HSOs often include billing, IT, marketing, human resources, payroll and accounting.

These organizations may or may not have doctor/advisors on their staff. Understand that these organizations exist as business entities for profit and are not healthcare providers, per se.

There are similarities in the transaction of selling a practice to an HSO compared to that of a traditional sale; there are also differences. Since the purchase price will be determined by reports similar to what a traditional buyer would require, you need to show up with the best possible set of financial statements and reports and have your practice in order and running at peak production, revenue and profitability to sell it for the best price.

In most cases, however, the HSO will want the original doctor/owner to stay with the practice as a treatment provider after the sale is complete for a period of at least two years. The original owner/doctor will no longer be an owner or a partner. The former owner/doctor becomes an employee of the HSO.[65]

If the doctor didn't like the business part of ownership, in the HSO scenario, the responsibilities of managing the practice and the responsibilities of ownership will be in the hands of the HSO. Keep in mind, however, that the absence of managerial responsibilities does not also apply to more time off from treatment for the doctor. The caveat is that even though the owner/doctor will be giving up ownership and financial control of the practice, that doctor will be expected to produce the same dollar amounts or more as when he/she owned the practice.

Why would an owner/doctor consider this option since he/she will give up control but still work hard seeing patients? As stated above, this is for the owner who wants to get cash now before retiring from practicing, who enjoys practicing because he loves treating patients, and who does not want the responsibilities involved in financial management, staff management, insurance and billing headaches, etc. For the

---

[65] Rincon, Todd. Dentistry IQ. April 8, 2015.

owner/doctor with this mindset, this scenario can be a very lucrative alternative to an outright sale and forced retirement.

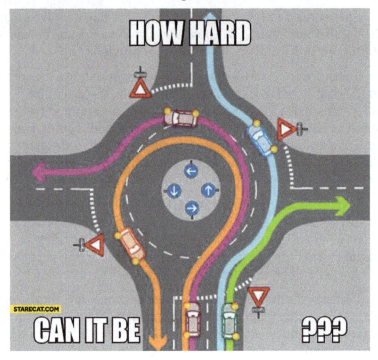

CHAPTER 25: HOW INVOLVED IS THE SELLING PROCESS

It is extremely important to understand that the normal selling process takes time to develop. The following illustrates the steps required to sell a practice. This is also what a potential buyer and seller should look for in the process. The summarized pathway for a sale looks something like this.[66]

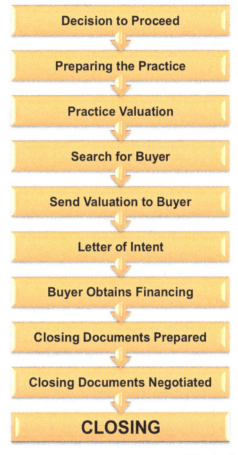

Decision to Proceed

Preparing the Practice

Practice Valuation

Search for Buyer

Send Valuation to Buyer

Letter of Intent

Buyer Obtains Financing

Closing Documents Prepared

Closing Documents Negotiated

CLOSING

©Tracker Enterprises, Inc.

[66]Hill, Roger K. *Transitions*. American Dental Association. 2006.

Selling Process Overview

The following individuals or teams will most likely be involved:

- Investment banker, broker/intermediary
- Accountants
- Attorneys
- Valuation professionals
- Transition experts
- The buyer
- The seller
- The lender
- Employees
- Other third parties

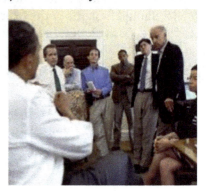

Create a process checklist

- Generate time lines
- Identify responsibilities and deadlines
- Start to set expectations

Create a sales process timeline

- A sample of steps and processes are described on the spreadsheet on the next page. *This is for illustration only*.
- Times to complete steps are optimistic estimates only; times can vary per step and may be longer than shown.
- When attorneys and accountants get involved in preparing the necessary information, time lines can easily be much longer.
- This is to help both the buyer and the seller estimate the time to completion and the complexity of the process.
- Note that the TOTAL WEEKS to complete on the sample timeline are less than the individual weeks estimated since many of the processes overlap each other.

Sales Process Timeline	Weeks to Complete
1 Initial meetings to determine deal strategy and expectation	1
2 Collect client (seller) data	2
3 Create a Confidential Business Report (CBR)	4
4 Initial contact with potential buyers and research buyers	7
5 Submit NDAs (Non-Disclosure Agreements) for signatures	5
6 Send CBR to interested buyers	4
7 Answer questions and solicit offers from interested parties	7
8 Perform initial DD (Due Diligence) with interested parties	6
9 Negotiate terms and offers with preferred buyers	5
10 Finalize and sign LOI (Letter of Intent) with preferred buyer	2
11 Provide exclusivity to buyer; buyer performs DD	7
12 Prepare DD information	24
13 Prepare legal documents to effect the sale	9
14 Close	1
TOTAL WEEKS	**30**

Definitions:

- **Confidential Business Reports (CBRs)**: Any business documents (e.g., P&Ls, Balance Sheets, etc.) that are to be kept secret and divulged to no one but the potential buyer and his/her advisors.

- **Non-Disclosure (NDA)/Confidentiality Agreement (CA)**: An NDA/CA is a contract by which one or more parties agree not to disclose confidential information, whether written or verbal, that they have shared as a part of doing business together.

- **Due Diligence (DD)**: This is the research and appraisal of a business undertaken by a prospective buyer, especially to establish its assets and liabilities and evaluate its commercial potential.

- **Letter of Intent (LOI)**: A document outlining the general plans of an agreement between two or more parties before a legal agreement is finalized. A LOI is not a contract and cannot be legally enforced; however, it signifies a serious commitment from one party to another.[67] This protects the seller from "shopping the deal."

---

[67] BusinessDictionary.com

171

Things you need to remember

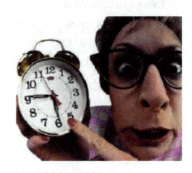

- Time is the enemy of all deals. A buyer's perception of your practice's value goes down and not up as time progresses.
- Address negatives first, then address positives later.
- Sellers loose their leverage to negotiate after the execution of the Letter of Intent.
- Consider all buyers because the appearance of "deep pockets" does not always make a good buyer.
- Remember, you are not selling yourself; you're selling the practice. The buyer must believe the practice can run independent of you.
- As the buyer's perception of risk decreases, value increases.
- If you want to or are asked by the buyer to stay post-sale, you will have to decide whether you want to do that. Reasons include:
  - Being available (e.g., 3 months), to introduce the new owner to patients. This is often part of the sale at no additional charge.
  - Staying on as an employee to handle high patient volume. Compensation is usually based on hourly, salary, or percentage of production or revenue associated with your performance.

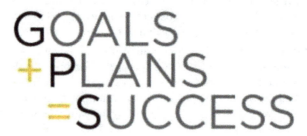

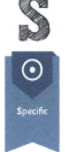   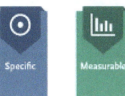 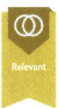 

All goals must be SMART

- **S**pecific
- **M**easurable
- **A**ttainable (i.e., **A**chievable)
- **R**elevant and **R**ealistic
- **T**ime-based and **T**ime-bound

Both buyer and seller have goals

Goals for the buyer ...

- Retention of the patient base
- Maintaining or improving production, revenue, and expenses
- Retention of key employees (e.g., office manager, etc.)
- Ability to perform existing services
- Protection including a Covenant Not To Compete

Questions for the Seller ...

- Do you want to sell and exit?
- Do you want to continue in the practice? (e.g., an employee)
- Do you want to diversify risk? (e.g., bring on a partner)
- Do you want to transfer the business to a hired associate(s)?

Do You Need an Attorney?

Both seller and buyer need to have excellent legal advice. The attorney's roles in the deal are as follows:

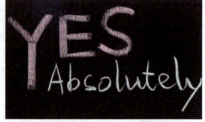

- **The attorney does not represent "the deal." The attorney represents <u>either</u> the buyer or the seller.**
- Manages the deal on behalf of the seller or buyer such as:
  - Identifies key business, legal, financing and tax issues.
  - Identifies the specific risks for each deal.
  - Manages the process and interpersonal dynamics of the deal with the client, intermediary, opposing party, etc.
- Role of the seller's attorney
  - Prepares the client for the deal process
  - Counsels the client on deal points
  - Assists in preparing and reviewing the due-diligence
  - Reviews and negotiates all transaction documents
    - o Confidentiality Agreement
    - o Letter of Intent
    - o Acquisition Agreements
  - Finds solutions to close the deal
- Role as buyer's attorney
  - Prepares the client for the deal process
  - Counsels the client on deal points
  - Conducts and coordinates legal due diligence
  - Prepares, reviews and negotiates all documents
  - Finds solutions to close the deal
- Choose an attorney who has advised healthcare professionals in your healthcare field before and who has a history of good results in negotiating practice purchases and sales.

Choose the vendor (attorney) that best matches your identity. And, if they don't have the scars, they don't have the wisdom.

The provisions of the deal ...

How will the purchase price be allocated?

- **All cash**. Buyer uses personal, friends' or relatives' cash or buyer obtains cash from a lending party (preferred since Seller gets all cash and assumes no personal risk).
- **Deferred purchase arrangement or seller financing**. Seller agrees to a promissory note that allows purchase over a specified period of time and interest rate. This contains:
  - Personal guarantees from the buyer
  - A possible balloon payment at a certain future date
  - A clause stating seller gets consideration if buyer defaults e.g., ownership of the practice returns back to seller, etc.
- **Stock** as a portion of the purchase price (only for C-Corporations); this can be VERY lucrative to Seller and Buyer. Seller avoids significant taxation for gains from sale; Buyer can negotiate a lower sales price since Seller decreases taxes.
- **Earnouts**: This is a performance-based component of the final price. It is a method of triggering increases in the purchase price based upon the future performance of the buyer. It can resolve issues regarding the purchase price:
  - Bridges gap between buyer's price (based on historical results) and seller's price (based on projected earnings).
  - Resolves differences of opinions on the valuation target.[68]

Other provisions/addendums might include:

- Covenant Not to Compete
- Non-Solicitation of Staff and/or Patients

An in depth explanation of how to prepare for a practice sale or purchase is beyond the scope of this book. If you would like help preparing, ask me about what we offer and how we can help you by emailing me at pjp@trackerenterprises.com.

---

[68] Blees, Chris. *To Sell Your Business*. Biggs-Kofford. 2015. No longer available.

Sell Summary:

1. When is the best time to prepare your practice to sell?
2. Do you have a transition plan in place?
3. Will there be a market for your practice? Understanding the current market conditions:
   a. Seller/Purchaser ratios
   b. Demographics
   c. Planning time frames
   d. Marketing the practice
4. How to protect yourself and family
   a. Establish goals
   b. Measure, monitor and evaluate
   c. Maximize the practice value
   d. Create a transition team
   e. Ensure business continuity
5. What is a Practice Valuation and what should it include?
6. Steps for arriving at a value for your practice include
   a. Choosing a valuation method
      i. Discounted Cash Flow
      ii. Excess Earnings including Goodwill
      iii. Multiple of Discretionary Earnings
   b. Items needed for the valuation process
7. Understanding Value Drivers and Value Killers
8. Considering alternatives to outright retirement (HSOs)
9. Understanding the steps involved in the selling process
10. Who should be on your selling team?
11. Creating a selling process checklist
12. Creating a selling process timeline
13. Understanding the definitions involved in the selling process
14. Understanding goals and questions
    a. Goals for the buyer
    b. Questions for the seller

Sell Action Plan: The Road Map

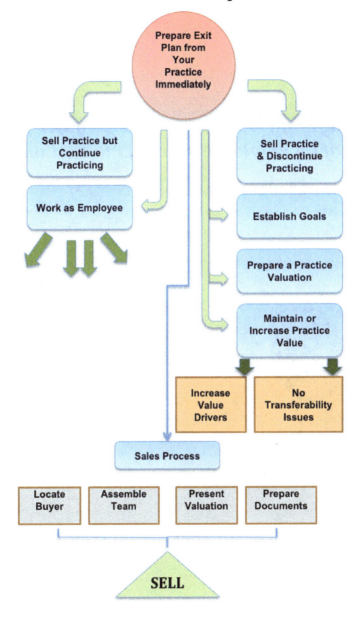

A fulfilling job experience is a major part of an employee's [your] motivation.

Shep Hyken

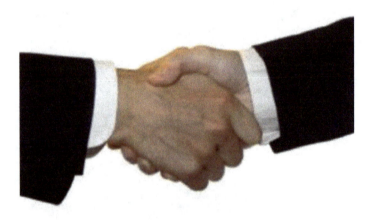

SECTION VI: SHOULD YOU WORK FOR SOMEONE ELSE?

If you do not want to immediately (or ever) pursue ownership of a practice, but you want to provide healthcare services to patients who can benefit from your expertise, you should not feel as if you are a second-class healthcare provider, unmotivated, or a failure simply because you want to be someone else's employee.

CHAPTER 26: EMPLOYMENT OPTIONS

You may be considering or have already committed to an employment position. This scenario might apply to any of the following employment opportunities:

- **Military**: This includes healthcare professionals obligated to a specific amount of time in the military due to a previous ROTC commitment, a military scholarship, or an enlistment commitment. The bonuses, guaranteed pay, scholarships, specialty training, continuing education, travel, hours, etc. can be really inviting reasons to choose this option. The negatives include having no wiggle room with the "employment" contract, the likelihood that your family will be uprooted often during your career, and pay that is usually less than you might realize in private practice or associateships.

- **Associateship (Employee)**: This option usually indicates you will be working for another practice owner or in a corporate structure (examples hospitals, corporate practices, HSOs, etc.). These options usually have the benefits of included health coverage, disability, life and malpractice insurance, savings and retirement programs, paid time off, and reasonably good incomes without the headaches of ownership. Negatives include having to work for someone else, a pay scale that could be lower than often seen in private practices, having contracts that include undesirable work schedules, covenants not to compete if you resign or are terminated, etc.

CHAPTER 27: RELATIONSHIP CONCERNS

What to consider before becoming an employee

1. The owner must have the patient flow to support an associate. Until the practice has more patients than it can handle, or if you (the associate) bring treatment options that are in great demand by the practice's patients that only you can provide, don't consider the position.
2. If the practice is experiencing growth, consider the position.
3. If the owner wants to reduce treatment time, an associate can aid in this process. For example, if the owner would like to reduce treatment by a day or more per week, an associate can take his place in order to maintain or enhance production. In addition, if the owner wants to maximize the treatment time available since he is paying for an office space 24/7, an associate can add additional treatment time.
4. The owner may also want to limit the scope of the services he provides. For example, the owner may want to limit exposure to a specific range of services, but the practice has a large number of patients who need these services. A qualified associate can continue to provide those services without loss of revenue. The associate may be qualified in requested procedures that the owner does not provide; adding these services can further enhance production and revenue.
5. The owner may be at the point in his/her career when the owner wants to start preparing for a transition, i.e., a future sale of the practice. One way to do this is to bring on an associate with a buy-in possibility. The associate should request a First Right of Refusal, a legal document that indicates that if the owner opts to sell, the associate has an option to buy before any one else; if the associate declines to enter into the transaction, the owner is then free to open the bidding up to other interested parties.[69]

---

[69] Investopedia.
https://www.investopedia.com/terms/r/rightoffirstrefusal.asp#ixzz5Fxv4NZDK

What can ruin an associate/owner relationship

Personality. There may be personality conflicts that can cause the relationship to fail. A good way to evaluate each other is to meet for dinner – include the spouses. Remember that although each party will be working with each other, the spouses will probably be the closest advisors. Be certain all parties are comfortable. Another way to determine

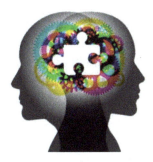

personality traits is to invite each other to a sports outing, e.g. golf. If either party "cheats a little" while playing, chances are this trait will carry through to future interactions.

1. **Transition Opportunities**. If the associate is interested in pursuing future ownership of the practice, preparing a transition plan between the parties can provide assurance that the associate will have first right of refusal when the owner decides to sell the practice.[70]

> A **First Right of Refusal** is a contractual right granted by an owner. The owner gives the holder of the right an opportunity to enter into a business transaction with the owner according to specified terms, before the owner may enter into that transaction with a third party.

2. **Planning Failure**. The most common reasons for failure are unfulfilled expectations. Comprehensive planning should define expectations in three areas:

    a. Expected economic outcomes
    b. Legal rights and obligations
    c. Sequencing of proper steps

---

[70] Frank, Brady. *The DDSO: Dentist-Owned Private Group Models*. Dental Economics, October 2017.

CHAPTER 28: UNDERSTANDING THE ASSOCIATE CONTRACT

Handshakes and verbal agreements are ancient history; don't repeat history. The associate should receive a copy of the written employment agreement and be permitted to take it to legal counsel for advice. <u>If you are not given this opportunity, decline the employment offer</u>. All contracts should be negotiable.

The following represents sections in a typical associate agreement. Each section demonstrates points and concerns that need to be considered by each of the parties and their attorneys.

1. **Introduction**: It defines
    a. Name and address of practice owner (called "Corporation" from this point forward).
    b. Name of the employee doctor (called "Doctor" from this point forward).
2. **Recitals**: This paragraph defines that the
    a. Doctor is legally licensed to practice (dentistry, medicine, etc.) in the state of employment.
    b. Corporation should request a copy of Doctor's state license prior to any further negotiations.
3. **Employment**:
    a. Doctor agrees to work only in Corporation's practice(s).
    b. Doctor agrees to perform duties assigned (or assigned in the future) by Corporation.
    c. Doctor agrees to abide by Employee Handbook.

> Associate should request to see Employee Handbook before signing Agreement and be permitted to have his attorney review it.

    d. Doctor agrees not to treat any patients (in any other practice) without written approval by Corporation.
    e. All revenue received for treatment remains the property of the Corporation.
    f. Doctor will do all that is required by Agreement and will not violate anything that might compromise the Corporation ethics or the legal requirements of the professional societies, federal, state or municipal laws.

4. **Term**: Indicates the official start date for Doctor. It specifies date on which all compensation, benefits, etc. will be based. It outlines reasons and when Doctor can be terminated.

    a. Termination of Employment. There is usually a notice provision that should be identical for both parties. If the Corporation does not want the Doctor to continue to render services during the notice period before the actual termination date, the Doctor should continue to be paid until the termination date.

    > It is recommended that associate read **Employment-At-Will** information in Chapter 7 since this Term paragraph may include an at will employment clause. **At will employment** allows Corporation or Doctor to end the Agreement for employment without notice or cause.

    b. Termination for cause or a material breach by Corporation (e.g., failure to pay compensation) provides for termination. Immediate termination also occurs upon Doctor's death, disability, for loss of license, etc.[71]

5. **Compensation**: Compensation should state whether it is based on an hourly, daily, weekly or monthly salary, or a percentage of collections or production.

    a. If employment terminates and

    > While compensation as a percentage of collections is common, a percentage of production is preferred because the associate cannot control the collection policy of the practice or the employees who process patient payments and insurance copayments. A base salary plus a % of production after a predetermined production minimum can be a great incentive for the associate.

---

[71] Prescott, William, Esq., "The Associate Contract". Dental Economics. May 2017.

compensation is based on collections, include a provision that compensation will continue for a period, e.g., 120 days, to allow for fees to be collected along with monthly accounting.

> The most common compensation is 30% for general practitioners and 35%-plus for specialists in addition to benefits, direct business expenses, and insurances for full-time associates.

b. If production is used, then compensation could be based on a percentage of usual and customary fee production or based on a percentage of adjusted production (*e.g., PPO fees*).

c. If bonuses are designated, bonuses are usually in the form of a reward for exceeding a predetermined level of production or collections. (*The formula needs to be included in the Agreement. Other bonuses might include signing, relocation, and student loans, provided that Doctor remains with the practice for a predetermined period of time.*)

> BE AWARE: If the agreements states that the associate's compensation is based on "adjusted production," this means that compensation could be reduced by any or all of the following: discounts, reduced fees, insurance and other write-offs, laboratory remakes, and uncollectable accounts. If there is a reduction, the percentage is increased and the formula should be adjusted production or collections, less the lab percentage, multiplied by the commission percentage. Remember that you should not be responsible for the collection policies and insurance plans accepted by the Owner/Corporation.

6. **Benefits**: All benefits are at the discretion of Corporation and should be spelled out in the EMPLOYEE HANDBOOK. (*Part-time employees usually do not receive benefits.*)
   a. Holidays: Average is 6-8 paid holidays per year. The usual paid holidays include New Year's Day, Easter, Memorial Day, July 4, Labor Day, Thanksgiving, and Fridays after Thanksgiving and Christmas (only if Christmas falls on a Thursday). *If Doctor comes in for emergencies on a holiday, be certain that it is stated in the agreement how Doctor will be paid.*
   b. Vacation: Average vacation time for associates after one year of service is 10 days. This is mandated by Corporation and is not subject to federal or state laws.
   c. Personal Days: This provides for paid or unpaid time off for each 12 months of the employment term. The time off is typically non-cumulative and forfeited if not taken with the applicable period. The time off may not interfere with the practice owner's scheduled time off and adequate advance notice must be provided, typically no less than 30 days. Time off should need to be approved in advance by Corporation. Other time off is typically unpaid. The average personal days offered are 2 – 6 days per year.
   d. Continuing Education: This will show how many days per year will be allowed to attend professional seminars, etc. It will indicate the annual allowance covered by Corporation for continuing education and whether that allowance can be carried over to the

next year. *Check if certain CE courses are required by the Corporation or whether courses chosen are Doctor's choice. Also check for who pays for lodging, meals, and transportation. Is overtime paid if it occurs?*

e. Health Insurance: This will designate who is covered (e.g., Doctor, Doctor and immediate family, etc.), when eligibility starts, etc.

f. Life Insurance: What is the life insurance benefit amount, if any? Who chooses the beneficiary?

g. Long-Term Disability Insurance: How much will premiums be, when are premiums due (annually, semi-annually, quarterly), how much are monthly disability payments, will insurance payouts be taxable (*remember that if premiums are paid by Corporation, taxation will apply*), and what age do benefits end? Will premiums be shared or not?

h. Professional Liability Insurance: Doctor must carry professional liability insurance. Doctor's policy should cover the practice as a "named" insured.

7. **Work Schedule**: If the employment is full-time, the specific days and times should be designated in a schedule in the agreement. If employment is part-time, the days and times are still designated, but a provision may state, "Doctor's workdays shall be increased or decreased in accordance with Corporation's need."[72]

> An employer is responsible to pay overtime for all employees, whether they are hourly or salaried.

a. Corporation is required to pay overtime (1½ times hourly rate) anytime Doctor works more than 9 hours in any one day or more than 40 hours in any one week.

b. *Be certain that Corporation pays overtime when regular hours plus on-call emergency hours are over 40 hours per week.*

---

[72] Prescott, William, Esq., "The Associate Contract". Dental Economics. May 2017.

8. **Performance and Salary Review**: What a review covers.
    a. Ask about what criteria are used to determine future bonuses, benefits and salary increases.
    b. Reviews should be no less than once per year, *but a newer, more preferred method is to schedule short reviews (e.g., once per month) to share information about performance, expectations, and goals. This way Doctor knows how he/she is performing.*
9. **Office Facilities**: This indicates that Corporation will furnish Doctor with office, laboratory, x-ray and other facilities, equipment, supplies, and ancillary personnel to enable Doctor to perform Doctor's duties on behalf of Corporation.
10. **Expenses**: This section indicates
    a. Who is financially responsible for continuing education and other Corporation-required programs?
    b. It should stipulate that if courses are required by Corporation, then all travel, meal, and lodging expenses will be covered by Corporation.
    c. If Doctor opts for Doctor's own preferred continuing education course, is Corporation responsible for expenses and for how much?
11. **Patient Records/Solicitation of Patients**: This is often part of the Non-Solicitation/Non-Compete/Restrictive Covenants section of the agreement or in an addendum to the agreement. This protects confidential information such as patient and referral source lists, noncompetition within a geographic radius or attached map, and, for a period of time (e.g., usually 1-3 years), non-solicitation of patients and/or referral sources and non-solicitation of staff members.
    a. The non-solicitation of patients, referral sources, and staff should be in effect immediately. Patients directly referred to the practice by Doctor, as well as the Doctor's friends and family (referred to as "Doctor's patients") should be excluded from the restrictive covenant provisions. Should Doctor's employment terminate, charts and records of Doctor's friends and family remain Doctor's property, unless Doctor chooses to have records remain with Corporation.

b. The Corporation should be responsible to notify the patients of Doctor if Doctor leaves the practice. Doctor should not agree to any requirement to testify in any proceeding following employment termination not involving Doctor. Doctor should be sure to have records

> Associates should not be required to write a letter to patients the associate previously treated that recommends those patients remain with the practice when the associate leaves.

access, at a "reasonable cost," if an attorney needs to defend Doctor in a lawsuit or proceeding.

c. If the contract includes an indemnification or hold harmless provision, Doctor should hold harmless or indemnify Corporation for any act causing liability not covered by insurance and vice versa.[73]

12. **Non-solicitation of Employees**: This stipulates that during the period of Doctor's employment and for a period of time (*e.g., the standard is 18 months*) after the end of employment, whether with or without cause, Doctor will not solicit any current or former employee of Corporation to leave employment or to work for Doctor at another location.

13. **Confidentiality Information**: This protects Corporation and Doctor from unduly disclosing confidential information.

14. **Specific Performance**: Both parties agree that if any controversy concerning the rights or obligations under this agreement arises, those rights or obligations will be enforceable in a court of law.

15. **Assignment**: This indicates that the rights, interests and benefits cannot be assigned, transferred, or pledged.

16. **Notice**: This indicates that any and all notices or any other communications will be given in writing by registered or certified mail, return receipt requested, and will include the addresses of both parties. It will also state the responsibility

---

[73] Prescott, William, Esq., "The Associate Contract". Dental Economics. May 2017.

of the Doctor to keep the Corporation informed of the Doctor's home telephone number, cell phone number and current home address.

17. **Governing Law**: This indicates the agreement will be subject to the laws of a state (usually the state of the location of the practice).

18. **Entire Agreement**: This simply states this is the entire agreement and will contain the signatures of both parties.

If a restrictive covenant is included with a minimum mileage radius, the mileage may vary depending on Corporation office location. For example, "urban" mileage maximums may be from 1-3 miles while "rural" and "agricultural" locations may be significantly higher at 10-25 miles.

Do not agree to geographic restrictions for multiple or future locations. If the associate grew up or resides in the geographic area where the practice is located, a buyout of the restrictive covenant can be an effective option.

An in depth discussion on associate contracts is beyond the scope of this book. Let me help you prepare for your employment agreement with your potential employer. If you need help with further clarification or if you need extra help understanding whether your employment agreement is in your best interest, ask me about what we offer and how we can help you by emailing me at pjp@trackerenterprises.com.

Don't be a square peg in a round hole.
The IRS doesn't like it.

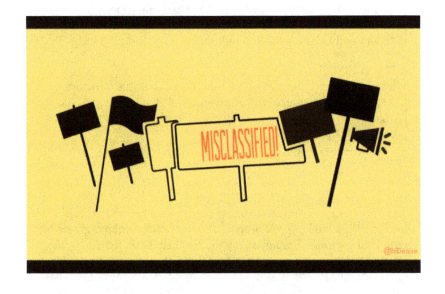

Chapter 29: Independent Contractor – Beware

Understand the definitions first ...

An **employee** is a person hired for a wage, salary, fee or payment to perform work for an employer. Generally, the employer must withhold income taxes, withhold and pay Social Security and Medicare taxes, and pay unemployment tax on wages paid to an employee. The first step is to complete IRS Form W-4.

An **independent contractor** is a person who contracts to do work for another person according to his or her own processes and methods; the contractor is not subject to another's control except for what is specified in a mutually binding agreement for a specific job. This person or business performs services for another person or entity under a contract between them, with the terms spelled out such as duties, pay, the amount and type of work and other matters.[74] To validate this arrangement, the first step is to have the contractor complete IRS Form W-9.

Healthcare people such as dentists, hygienists, physicians, chiropractors, veterinarians, etc., who either own their businesses or whose services are for hire, are often faced with questions relating to independent contractorship. Employees and individual contractors often have a huge misconception of the Federal government's view of individual contractors in the employment marketplace.

Due to recent increased interest by the IRS, it is now more important than ever that business owners and their workers understand the government's position. The IRS is viewing the increased usage of contractors with more suspicion than ever. The IRS estimates it loses $1.5 billion annually in income, Social Security, and unemployment tax revenue from misclassifying workers as independent contractors. The misclassification costs

---

[74] Gerald and Kathleen Hill. *The People's Law Dictionary*. Fine Communications.

are estimated to cost $8.71 billion for the periods of fiscal years 2012 through 2021.[75]

The question as to whether individuals are employees or independent contractors depends on the facts in each case. The general rule is that an individual is an independent contractor if the business owner has the right to control or direct only the result of the work and not the means and methods of accomplishing the result.[76]

Advantages to Employers and Contractors

Workers often prefer to be reclassified as independent contractors because they can fully offset benefits against income and receive a higher rate of compensation (at least that's the conception that the independent contractor hopes the employer will do for them) since the employer has eliminated payroll taxes and benefit costs.

Employers achieve their objective of reducing labor costs (direct wages and employee benefits) by either hiring workers as independent contractors or terminating existing employees and rehiring them as independent contractors. An advantage of labeling a worker as an independent contractor is that it lowers an employer's tax obligation since the employer does not have to pay the independent contractor's Federal Insurance Contribution Act (FICA) or Federal Unemployment Tax Act (FUTA) taxes. In addition, the employer is not required to provide employee benefits (e.g., workers' compensation insurance, vacation, sick leave, health insurance, pension contributions, etc.).

---

[75] National Employment Law Project, Fact Sheet, 2015.

[76] IRS Publication 15-A. Employer's Supplemental Tax Guide. 2017.

Disadvantages for Independent Contractors

The disadvantages to the independent contractors include denying them the protection of workplace laws and the absence of unemployment insurance and workers' compensation. Independent contractors are responsible for paying their own estimated taxes.

How the IRS defines an Independent Contractor

The IRS focuses on the concept of who is in control. Ruling 87-41 states that: *"Generally, the relationship of employer and employee exists when the person for whom the services are performed has the right to control and direct the individual who performs the services not only as to the result to be accomplished by the work, but also as to the details and means by which that result is accomplished. That is, an employee is subject to the will and control of the employer not only as to what shall be done but as to how it shall be done."*

Ruling 87-41 lists a twenty-question test that the IRS uses in determining the correct worker's classification status (see bold print in itemized points below). Employers can use these factors in evaluating their own workforces to determine if workers are appropriately classified. These IRS questions are:

1. **Is the worker subject to the employer's instructions?** A worker who is required to comply with the employer's instructions as to when, where and how work is to be done is most likely an employee. It is only required that an employer have the right to control the worker; the control implemented is irrelevant.
2. **Does the employer provide training?** Any form of employer-provided training suggests an employee-employer relationship since training implies that the work needs to be performed in a particular manner.
3. **What is the degree of integration of the services?** If the success of the services performed by the worker is crucial to the success of the business, control over the services is presumed to exist.

4. **Does the worker personally render the services?** Services required by the employer indicate employer control.
5. **Who is responsible for hiring, supervising and paying?** Hiring, directing, or paying, when done by the employer, shows an employee-employer arrangement.
6. **Does a continuing relationship exist?** Continuing work by the individual, even if not regular, points toward an employer-employee relationship.
7. **Does the employer set hours of work?** If the employer designates work hours, this demonstrates control over the worker.
8. **Is full-time work required?** Utilizing a worker on a full-time basis precludes the worker from pursuing other work and is an indication of control.
9. **Is the person doing work on the employer's premises?** This tends to indicate control by the employer and is indicative of employment status.
10. **Is the work order or sequences set by the employer?** Following routines or work patterns established by the employer is indicative of employee status.
11. **Are oral/written reports required?** The requiring of regular progress reports demonstrates control.
12. **Is payment by the hour, week or month?** Payment on a fixed periodic basis, rather than upon completion of the work, is an indicator of employee status.
13. **Does the employer make payment for business and/or traveling expenses?** The payment of these expenses by the employer points to regulation of business activities and indicates employee status.
14. **Is the employer responsible for the furnishing of tools and materials?** Independent contractors normally provide their own tools and materials.
15. **Is the worker required to make a significant investment to perform the work?** The making of an investment by the worker, e.g. rental of a facility, supports the existence of independence as an independent contractor.

16. **Does performance result in realization of profit or loss?** The ability to realize either a profit or a loss in performing the work is a characteristic of an independent contractor.
17. **Is the individual working for more than one firm at a time?** The performance of services for several customers simultaneously is typical of an independent contractor.
18. **Is the individual engaged in making service available to the general public?** Marketing one's services to the general public indicates independence.
19. **Does the employer have a unilateral right to discharge the worker?** The right to discharge at will indicates an employer-employee relationship. Independent contractors typically can only be discharged for failure to meet contract requirements.
20. **Does the worker have a unilateral right to terminate his services?** An employee may resign at will, but an independent contractor may be contractually obligated to perform.

The consequences of misclassifying workers

An employer should also be aware that each time he files the required Form 1099-MISC for payments to an independent contractor, it is providing notice to the IRS of having a work relationship with an independent contractor. In addition, there is always the possibility that a disgruntled independent contractor will later allege that an employer-employee relationship existed in an attempt to hold the employer liable for withholding and payroll taxes.

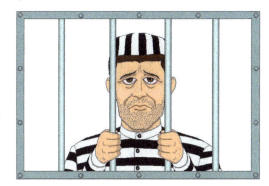

The Revenue Reconciliation Act provides for monetary penalties for negligent disregard of the tax rules and regulations. Employer assessments may apply such as: (1) interest on tax underpayments is payable to IRS, compounded daily, (2) the employer share of FICA tax of the worker's pay and additional tax for the worker's share of FICA and Medicare taxes, (3) additional tax for the worker's Federal withholding taxes, (4) FUTA taxes, (5) the bill for IRS back taxes and related penalties and interest of the employee's back pay, (6) criminal penalties may be enforced, (7) additional add-on penalty interest expenses, and (8) independent contractors may sue their employers and collect for unwithheld taxes. In addition, the IRS may notify the appropriate state governmental taxing authority and a corresponding state unemployment audit may follow.[77]

Maybe you've never thought much about the difference between being an independent contractor or an employee or being an employer and having a work relationship with one. If you are accepting a worker as an independent contractor, you should know the key differences. The IRS consequences involved in not knowing can be significant and severe.

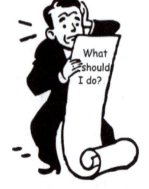

Whether you are offering your services to an employer or whether you are an employer, don't gamble with your future. If you have additional questions about the laws regarding independent contractors, speak with an experienced employment attorney and your accountant today.

---

[77] https://www.irs.gov/forms-pubs/RDA-2017-10-12-2017-Form-1096, http://www.irs.gov/publications/p15a/index.html, https://www.irs.gov/pub/irs-pdf/fss8.pdf

CHAPTER 30: DOES RENTING SPACE MAKE SENSE?

There is one more option

If you don't want to own or lease your own office and you don't want to work for someone else, you might consider renting space from another practitioner who might be interested in receiving rental income for space not being used.

Practitioners who have their own office space are paying for that space 24 hours a day, 7 days a week, and 365 days every year. They might have treatment rooms open during the other hours of the week. For example, I worked on Monday, Tuesday, 1/2 day on Wednesday, Thursday and then took the remainder of the week off. Therefore, Wednesday afternoons, Fridays and Saturdays were available for someone else to treat patients without that person getting in my way.

This schedule was especially attractive to specialists who wanted part-space in another part of town distant from their practices. It was also attractive to semi-retired practitioners who only wanted to work a few days each week. If all else failed, the renting practitioner could opt to see patients on those days and the evenings I did not work.

A rental agreement, including all verbiage to protect the owner, will need to be executed by the owner's attorney. It should indicate that the renting practitioner is liable for all patient treatment. If the renter uses any of the owner's equipment or staff, the owner should add to the base rent to cover any expenses (additional supplies used) that will cost the owner more. In addition, the renting practitioner should be financially responsible for any of the owner's equipment damaged or lost.

This arrangement can add dollars to the owner's monthly revenue without the owner taking on the liability burdens associated with employee practitioners. It gives the renter the advantage of having a space to practice without the higher costs associated with ownership.

Employment Summary:

1. Understand your potential employment options if you do not plan on currently or ever owning your own practice.
   a. Military
   b. Associateship (all other options as an employee)
2. What to look for before becoming someone else's employee
   a. Does the employer really need another employee?
   b. Avoiding problems before becoming an employee
3. Understanding the sections and interpreting an Associate Contract
   a. Introduction
   b. Recitals
   c. Employment
   d. Term
   e. Compensation and benefits
   f. Work Schedule
   g. Performance and Salary Reviews
   h. Office Facilities
   i. Expenses (who is responsible)
   j. Patient Records and Patient Solicitation
   k. Non-Solicitation of Employees
   l. Confidentiality Information
   m. Specific Performance
   n. Assignment
   o. Notice
   p. Governing Law
   q. Signatures, etc.
4. Independent Contractor status
   a. Are you considering work as an independent contractor
   b. Understand employee vs. independent contractor status
   c. What are the advantages and disadvantages
   d. How the IRS defines independent contractor status
   e. What are the consequence of misclassification
5. Option to rent another practitioner's space

Employment Action Plan: The Road Map

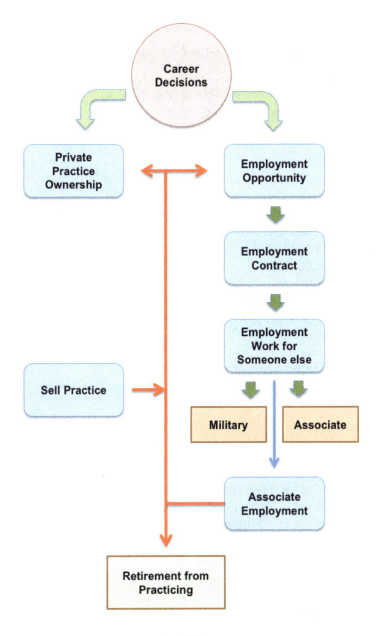

SECTION VII: IN A NUTSHELL

Seek to discover it, for it is this thread
that holds you to the past and binds you to the future.[78]

Section I – Does Leadership Make a Difference?

1. Understanding the basic concepts of leadership
2. The ideal Performance Management Process
   a. Philosophy & Purpose
   b. Goal setting
   c. Educating and coaching
   d. Observing
   e. Monitoring and measuring progress
   f. Meeting and updating frequently
   g. Praising and redirecting at all steps along the way
3. Why listening is so important
4. The Mutual Fussiness Factor
   a. Employer
   b. Employee
5. What options do you have when staff members resist?
6. The Employee Handbook's importance and what to include
   a. Legal policies
   b. Disclaimers
   c. All other items of importance
      i. Practice history and vision
      ii. Time-off policies
      iii. Employee behavior
      iv. Pay and promotions
      v. Benefits
      vi. Reasons for disciplinary action
      vii. Termination
      viii. Letter of Acknowledgement
7. Understanding "Employment at Will"
8. When and how to let an employee go

---

[78] Master Kan, Kung Fu, TV Series

Section II- Launch

1. Where are you now?
   a. Healthcare student
   b. Residency program
   c. Healthcare faculty
   d. Hospital staff
   e. Military
   f. Associate (employee)
   g. Practice owner
   h. Healthcare Service Organization employee
   i. Looking at retiring
2. Which of the following stages of your Business Life Cycle are you experiencing or preparing to enter?
   a. Launch
   b. Expand
   c. Optimize
   d. Sell
3. How well do you understand basic business principles?
4. What should you avoid to prevent failure?
   a. Poor planning
   b. Poor management
   c. Inadequate financing
   d. Poor location
   e. Increase competition
   f. Low production
   g. Not adapting to change
5. Obtaining sources of financing
6. Choosing the correct business structure
7. Advisory Team: Choose an experienced accountant and attorney.

Section III – Expand

1. Why you need to understand business principles.
2. Do you know:
   a. Where you are
   b. Where you're going
   c. Where you've been
3. What is the Optimal Business Management system?
   a. Planning
   b. Monitoring
   c. Analyzing
   d. Anticipating
   e. Improving
4. Consider monitoring these statistics:
   a. Production
   b. Revenue
   c. Accounts receivables
   d. Provider statistics
   e. Labor costs including salaries and benefits
   f. All expenses including debt service
   g. Scheduling
   h. Patient information statistics
5. The three job descriptions you have
   a. Entrepreneur
   b. Manager (Owner)
   c. Technician
6. Understanding business terminology
   a. Production
   b. Revenue
   c. Expenses
   d. Net Income
   e. Profit
   f. Cash Flow
7. Understanding financial reports
   a. Profit and Loss Statements (P&L)/Income Statements
   b. Balance Sheets
   c. General Ledgers
   d. Cash Flow Statements

Section IV – Optimize

1. Key functions of Optimal Business Management in your practice:
    a. Maintaining your bookkeeping system
    b. Information tools including ways to monitor, measure, and manage using Key Performance Indicators (KPIs)
2. Regardless of your choice, you need to be versed in business
    a. If you are planning on the military, you will enter into private or corporate practice after the military.
    b. If you are an employee, you need to understand business to be able to negotiate your worth.
    c. If you are in a specialty program, you may eventually go into private practice or work as an employee.
3. Questions to continually ask yourself:
    a. Is the practice experiencing unusual gains or losses?
    b. Are profits holding or improving?
    c. Are profits keeping pace with expenses?
    d. How does cash flow compare with profit?
    e. Are changes consistent with the growth needed?
    f. Are there any signs of financial distress?
    g. Are there any unusual assets and liabilities?
4. Why is a Budget necessary and how to prepare a Budget?
5. Why are Forecasts necessary and how to prepare a Forecast?

Section V – Sell

1. When is the best time to prepare your practice to sell?
2. Do you have a transition plan in place?
3. Will there be a market for your practice? Understanding the current market conditions:
    e. Seller/Purchaser ratios
    f. Demographics
    g. Planning time frames
    h. Marketing the practice
4. How to protect yourself and family
    a. Establish goals
    b. Measure, monitor and evaluate
    c. Maximize the practice value
    d. Create a transition team
    e. Ensure business continuity
5. What is a Practice Valuation and what should it include
6. Steps for arriving at a value for your practice include
    a. Choosing a valuation method
        i. Discounted Cash Flow
        ii. Excess Earnings including Goodwill
        iii. Multiple of Discretionary Earnings
    b. Items needed for valuation process
7. Understanding Value Drivers and Value Killers
8. Considering alternatives to outright retirement (HSOs)
9. Understanding the steps involved in the selling process
10. Who should be on your selling team?
11. Creating a selling process checklist
12. Creating a selling process timeline
13. Understanding the definitions involved in the selling process
14. Understanding goals
    a. Goals for the buyer
    b. Goals for the seller

Section VI – Would You Prefer to Work for Someone Else?

1. Understand your potential employment options if you do not plan on currently or ever owning your own practice.
   a. Military
   b. Associateship (all other options as an employee)
2. What to look for before becoming someone else's employee
   a. Does the employer really need another employee?
   b. Avoiding problems before becoming an employee
      i. Personality conflicts
      ii. Transitioning opportunities and concerns
      iii. Failure to plan
3. Understanding and interpreting an Associate Contract
   a. Introduction
   b. Recitals
   c. Employment
   d. Term
   e. Compensation
   f. Benefits
   g. Work Schedule
   h. Performance and Salary Reviews
   i. Office Facilities
   j. Expenses (who is responsible)
   k. Patient Records and Patient Solicitation
   l. Non-Solicitation of Employees
   m. Confidentiality Information
   n. Specific Performance
   o. Assignment
   p. Notice
   q. Governing Law
   r. Signatures, etc.
4. Independent Contractor status
   a. Are you considering work as an independent contractor
   b. Understand employee vs. independent contractor status
   c. What are the advantages and disadvantages
   d. How the IRS defines independent contractor status
   e. What are the consequences of misclassification?

*A dream written down with a date
becomes a GOAL.
A goal broken down into steps
becomes a PLAN.
A plan backed by ACTION
makes your dreams come true!*
Greg Reid

POSTSCRIPT

I ask you to ...

- Challenge all sources of production, revenue and expenses

- Make decisions not based on emotional whim or guesswork but on solid information & facts

- Operate your business not by managing to the budget, but by managing to forecasts & constantly changing trends.

You need to take responsibility for yourself and, until you do, you can't go forward. You must focus on where you're going and what you'd like to see happen, rather than having your eyes glued to the rearview mirror, looking back at what was done and who did it. It's time to take back your power.

Take control of your practice and your bottom line! Yes, knowledge equals power, but knowledge also equals success. Practices that successfully forecast their financial futures have a competitive edge.

Remember, success in only a short journey away. Follow these rules:

1. **Set clear goals, then MONITOR & MEASURE** performance.
2. **Your revenue has to exceed your expenses.**
3. **Collect your accounts receivables.** Don't be a banker.
4. **Take care of your customers.** Remember the Golden Rule: "*Do to others what you want them to do to you.*"
5. **Take care of your people.** Don't expect your employees to treat patients and vendors with respect and compassion if you don't treat your employees with respect and compassion.
6. **PRAISE progress**, even minimal progress, & REDIRECT inappropriate behavior.
7. **LISTEN, LISTEN, LISTEN.** Pay attention to what your patients and your staff are trying to relate to you.

Think in terms of going to the third power:

Always follow the three Ms:

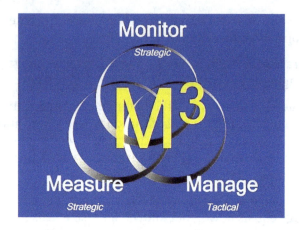

So that you can succeed with the three Ws:

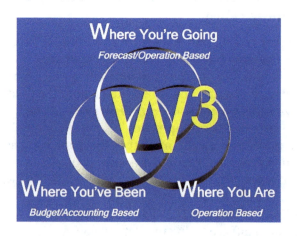

©Tracker Enterprises, Inc. 2018

If, after reading this book, you understand the concepts and reasons presented to justify your use of Business Life Cycle Management, but you have no desire or time to study and evaluate your financial information, I have a recommendation. Tracker Enterprises, Inc. can set up a customized program for your practice so that you can tell where you've been, where you are, and where you're going. We'll design an action plan specifically for your needs, and we'll ensure convenience, confidentiality and an on-going commitment to help you make your business goals a reality. If you need assistance or have questions, send me an email at pjp@trackerenterprises.com. Visit our website at www.trackerenterprises.com to view my Blogs, Podcasts, Seminars, Webinars, etc.

***ALL OUR DREAMS CAN COME TRUE
IF WE HAVE THE COURAGE TO PURSUE THEM.***

THANKS FOR READING

I wish you the absolute best! – Paul

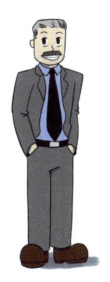

BIBLIOGRAPHY

American Heritage Dictionary. Dell Publishing, Inc., 1995.

American Heritage Dictionary. Houghton Mifflin, 2016.

Blanchard, Ken. The Heart of a Leader. Cook, 1999.

Blanchard & Hutson. *Full Steam Ahead*. Berrett-Koehler, 2003.

Blanchard & Hutson. *The One Minute Entrepreneur*. Berrett, 2004.

Blanchard & Johnson. *The One Minute Manager*. Harper-Collins, 2004.

Blanchard & Lorber. *Putting the One Minute Manager to Work*. Morrow, 1984.

Blanchard & Miller. *The Secret*. Berrett-Koehler, 2004.

Blees, Chris. *To Sell Your Business*. Biggs-Kofford. 2015.

Frank, Brady. *The DDSO: Dentist-Owned Private Group Models*. Dental Economics, October 2017.

Brandi, JoAnna. President, JoAnna Brandi & Company. 2006.

Brodsky, Norm. INC Magazine. June 2013.

Brown, John. Business Enterprise Institute. *Exit Planning Excuses*. 2017

BusinessDictionary.com

Candy, Frank. The Magic of Disney's Business Success. Discussions. April 2018.

Cardillo, Joseph. *Be Like Water*. Warner Books, Inc., 2003.

Carpenter, Gary. Personal Interviews & Discussions. 1990-2016.

Cohen, Allen. *The Portable MBA in Management*. Wiley, Inc., 1993.

Collins & Devanna. *The Portable MBA*. Wiley, Inc., 1992.

Connolly, Michael. Personal Discussions. 2004-2005.

Department of Commerce. https://www.commerce.gov/ .

Dictionary.com. www.dictionary.com/browse/crisis

Drucker, Peter. *Management.* Harper & Row, 1973.

Gerber, Michael. *The E Myth.* Harper Collings Publishers, 1995.

Gerber, Michael. *The E Myth Revisited.* Harper Collings, 2001.

Godin, Seth. *The Purple Cow.* The Penguin Group, 2003

Google. Advanced Image Search. https://www.google.com/advanced_image_search

Gostick & Telford. *The Integrity Advantage.* Gibbs-Smith, 2003.

Hall, Doug. *Jump Start Your Business Brain.* Brain Brew, 2001.

Hayes & Abernathy, *Harvard Business Review.*

Haywood, Aimee. Discussions. 2000-2001.

Hill, Gerald & Kathleen. *The People's Law Dictionary.* Fine Communications.

Hill, Roger K. *Transitions.* American Dental Association. 2006.

Khadem & Lorber. *One Page Management* William Morrow, 1986.

Investopedia. www.investopedia.com .

Lao-tzu. *Tao Te Ching.* CreateSpace, 2016. **ISBN-10:** 1535229330.

Lao-tzu. *Tao Te Ching. Kung Fu*, TV series, 1972-1975.

Klopp. *Idiot's Guide to Business Management.* Alpha Books, 1998.

Livingston, Gordon. *Too Soon Old Too Late Smart.* Marlowe, 2004.

Livingstone, John. *The Portable MBA.* Wiley & Sons, Inc., 1992.

Matthews, Gail. Psychology professor. Dominican University, California.

Merriam-Webster. https://www.merriam-webster.com/dictionary/crisis

Mercado, Darla. Your Money Your Future. CNBC. January 9, 2018.

Muhl, Charles J. Former economist with The Bureau of Labor Statistics

Nelson, Bob. *1001 Ways to Reward Employees*. Workman, 1994.

Niemann, Nick. *The Business Model Myth Solution*. 2014.

Pavlik, Beverly. Discussions. 1976-2018.

Peters, Tom. *A Passion for Excellence.* Warner Books, Inc., 1985.

Peters, Tom. *Design*. DK Publishing, Inc., 2005.

Peters, Tom. *Leadership*. DK Publishing, Inc., 2005.

Peters, Tom. *Re-imagine*. DK Publishing, Inc., 2003.

Peters, Tom. *Trends*. DK Publishing, Inc., 2005.

Potter, Terry, PhD. Discussions. Venture Solutions, 2001-2005.

Rincon, Todd. Dentistry IQ. April 8, 2015.

Roberts, Wess. *Victory Secrets of Attila the Hun*. Doubleday, 1993.

Ruger, Michael. Greenbush Financial Group, LLC. 2018.

Russell & Taylor. *Operations Management.* Prentice Hall, 1995.

Simon, Ruth. *The Wall Street Journal*. February 23, 2018.

Sletten, Paul. The Sletten Group. Denver, CO.

Smith, Mark S. A. Discussions. Bija Company, 2017-2018.

Smith, Mark S. A. Discussions, Outsource Channel Executives, Inc., 2000-2005.

Smith, Mark S. A. Executive Strategy Skills Summit. Bija Co, 2018.

Smith, Mark S. A. *From MSP to BSP, Pivot from Managed Service Provider to Business Services Provider to Profit from I.T. Disruption*, 2018.

Smith, Robert. Discussions. The Genimation Group. 2003-2005.

Stevens, Mark. *The 10-Minute Entrepreneur*. Warner, 1985.

Stiefler, Ken. *The Exit Planning Review*. Business Enterprises Inst. 2016.

Swanson, Boynton, Ross. *Accounting*, , SW Publishing, 1977.

Tatum, Doug. No Man's Land. The Penguin Group, 2008.

The Free Dictionary. Farlex. 2017.

The Small Business Sourcebook, Gale Publishing, 2004. ISBN-10: 1414479646

The Word for You Today. Celebration, Inc. 2018.

Tracy, John A. *Accounting for Dummies,* , Wiley Publishing, 2005.

Tyson & Schell. *Small Business for Dummies.* Wiley, Inc., 2003.

Van Fleet, James. *The 22 Biggest Mistakes Managers Make*. Parker Publ, 1973.

Wall Street Journal. 2017-2018.

Ward, Susan. *The Balance*.
https://www.thebalance.com/business-budget-2948312

Wells Fargo Works for Small Business, www.wellsfargo.com .

Wikipedia. www.wikipedia.com .

Yording, Chandra. Discussions. 2001-2006.

ABOUT THE AUTHOR

As a healthcare provider and business professional with more than 40 years experience, including practicing in the military and twenty-five years in private practice, Dr. Paul Pavlik has "walked the walk" and understands the daily and long-term responsibilities involved in running a healthcare practice. Paul is the founder and CEO of *Tracker Enterprises, Inc.* He established Tracker Enterprises, Inc. to help other healthcare professionals achieve financial success with 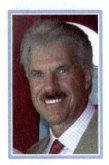 unique concepts and tools previously unavailable – tools that do not replace, but significantly augment, information received from an accountant, bookkeeper, financial consultant, and/or software management programs. Tracker Enterprises offers services and products, including a number of financial management tools and financial forecasting proprietary software that allow business owners to use sound Business Life Cycle Management concepts. Tracker consults with practices that have as few as two individuals to healthcare providers with over six hundred employees. Tracker Enterprises has earned the reputation of being part-time, off-site, or virtual CFOs these companies.

Paul is the chief consultant in charge of client relations and project management including writing business plans, preparing practice valuations, preparing entrance and exit strategies, brokering practice purchases and sales, evaluating and updating fee schedules, and interpreting financial reports resulting in Tracker's unique and proprietary monthly and yearly forecasting, budgeting, and "what if" scenarios. He feels that the variety of his experiences allows him to offer clients a "big picture" perspective without losing sight of the details. He enjoys helping healthcare providers and their staffs discover their direction and how their decisions affect them both now and into the future. His intention is to allow healthcare owners to understand their financials in one short session each month, to direct doctors on how to adjust their forecasting so that they can stay on track, and to make suggestions, where necessary, to allow them to meet or exceed their goals.

If your preference is to do all of the work yourself, we offer several options on training you and/or your team such as seminars, webinars and training modules.

If, however, you consider your time as a treatment provider too valuable to act as your own manager, we will be honored to work with you to manage your Business Life Cycle needs.

For more information on how we can help you better prepare for Business Life Cycle Management, contact us at pjp@trackerenterprises.com and visit our website at www.trackerenterprises.com.

CARICATURE ILLUSTRATIONS BY

Samuel A. Miller (SAM) is a freelance artist and illustrator who has experience in many media but specializes in character design. He is pursuing a degree in Art Education. He lives in a hobbit hole-like apartment with Rachael, who is his wife, friend and manager. His contact information follows:

Samuel A. Miller
Email: 4artstuff@gmail.com
Instagram: @sam_i_art
Website: Patreon.com/samuelamiller

Thank you, Sam, for doing such a wonderful job of preparing my caricature illustrations for this book. You are a real talent. I had a great experience working with you. - Paul

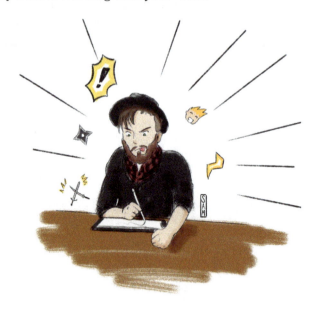

CPSIA information can be obtained
at www.ICGtesting.com
Printed in the USA
LVHW081415190321
681674LV00013B/1109